the
Eczema
diet

the Eczema diet

Discover how to stop &
prevent the itch of eczema
through diet & nutrition

Karen Fischer

Robert
ROSE

For complete cataloguing information, see page 259.

Disclaimer

This book is a general guide only and should never be a substitute for the skill, knowledge, and experience of a qualified medical professional dealing with the facts, circumstances, and symptoms of a particular case.

The nutritional, medical, and health information presented in this book is based on the research, training, and professional experience of the author, and is true and complete to the best of her knowledge. However, this book is intended only as an informative guide for those wishing to know more about health, nutrition, and medicine; it is not intended to replace or countermand the advice given by the reader's personal physician. Because each person and situation is unique, the author and the publisher urge the reader to check with a qualified health-care professional before using any procedure where there is a question as to its appropriateness. A physician should be consulted before beginning any exercise program. The author and the publisher are not responsible for any adverse effects or consequences resulting from the use of the information in this book. It is the responsibility of the reader to consult a physician or other qualified health-care professional regarding his or her personal care.

This book contains references to products that may not be available everywhere. The intent of the information provided is to be helpful; however, there is no guarantee of results associated with the information provided. Use of brand names is for educational purposes only and does not imply endorsement.

The recipes in this book have been carefully tested by our kitchen and our tasters. To the best of our knowledge, they are safe and nutritious for ordinary use and users. For those people with food or other allergies, or who have special food requirements or health issues, please read the suggested contents of each recipe carefully and determine whether or not they may create a problem for you. All recipes are used at the risk of the consumer. We cannot be responsible for any hazards, loss, or damage that may occur as a result of any recipe use. For those with special needs, allergies, requirements, or health problems, in the event of any doubt, please contact your medical adviser prior to the use of any recipe.

Caution: Before beginning the Eczema Diet, be sure to consult a medical doctor or a dermatologist. If you have medical conditions that are being treated with diet or drugs, follow the Eczema Diet with the supervision of your doctor or dietitian.

Design and Production: Daniella Zanchetta/PageWave Graphics Inc.
Editors: Bob Hilderley, Senior Editor, Health; and Sue Sumeraj, Recipes
Copy editor: Kelly Jones
Proofreader: Sheila Wawanash
Indexer: Gillian Watts
Cover image: Sliced papaya © iStockphoto.com/Lusoimages

Published by Robert Rose Inc.
120 Eglinton Avenue East, Suite 800, Toronto, Ontario, Canada M4P 1E2
Tel: (416) 322-6552 Fax: (416) 322-6936
www.robertrose.ca

Printed and bound in Canada

4 5 6 7 8 9 FP 21 20 19 18

*To appreciate the healing power of food,
you must first have something to heal.*

Contents

Preface

● ●

Itch Busters

First things first. The itch that best characterizes eczema is often so severe that you want to act immediately. Try these natural remedies and recipes at home when an itch attack occurs.

1. **Cold Compress:** Fill a sealable bag with ice cubes, wrap it in a towel, and hold it next to your itchy skin. For information on safe and effective topical skin care products, see "Beneficial Skin Care Ingredients," page 129.

2. **Baking Soda Bath:** Add baking soda to your bathwater. Immediately after bathing, use a towel to pat the skin until semi-dry. Then apply moisturizer to your entire body, and, if necessary, sparingly apply an ointment over the itchy areas. If you need more help, refer to the Bicarb Bath Recipe (page 136) and the emollients and moisturizers section (page 129).

3. **Alkalizing Drink:** Drink an alkalizing drink, such as Healthy Skin Juice, to decrease acidity in the body. Acid in the tissues can cause itchiness. Try making Tarzan Juice with added beets. Instead of a beverage, enjoy a serving of Alkaline Bomb Salad. For these recipes, see pages 206, 207, and 218, respectively.

4. **Nutrient Supplements:** Take magnesium, glycine, vitamin C, vitamin B6, and quercetin in supplement form. For dosage guidance, see "Top 15 Nutrient Supplements" for the total daily intakes for your age or your child's age (pages 95–123).

Introduction

My daughter Ayva was 2 weeks old when she developed spots on her face that resembled acne. The creases of her elbows and knees were red and weeping. When she was 10 months old, a nurse who had seen Ayva a few months earlier exclaimed, "Has your child still got eczema?" I thought what a rude comment that was. Eczema is a genetic condition, I had been told. What could I do about it? I had not considered treatment options for my baby beyond cortisone cream and thick ointments.

> Eczema is a genetic condition, I had been told. What could I do about it?

When Ayva was 1 year old, she was diagnosed with dust mite allergy, which meant she could no longer sleep with, or touch, any of her soft toys. We were advised to avoid junk food, additives, and salicylates. Playing on the grass, swimming in a pool, and petting the family cat inflamed Ayva's skin from head to toe. The cat was sent to Grandma's house and swimming lessons were canceled. Then one day, Ayva, who was growing resentful about being different from her friends, ate some food at a friend's birthday party, and her eczema spread farther down her legs. We noticed she was becoming more sensitive to everything. It was sad to see her suffering.

That was my incentive to begin researching eczema. By the time Ayva was 2 years old, I had devised a basic diet and supplement routine for her, and 2 months later, to my surprise, her eczema was gone. The temporary dietary changes were strict, but soon Ayva could enjoy normal activities, such as playing with fluffy toys and swimming in chlorinated pools. Occasionally, she could eat party food without her eczema returning, and she no longer needed topical steroids. Her diet was gradually expanded, and eventually she could eat all foods without her eczema returning.

At first glance, the Eczema Diet may seem like a regular elimination diet, but it differs in many ways. This diet is designed specifically for eczema sufferers. While on the Eczema Diet, you temporarily take problematic foods out of the diet and you eat nutritious eczema-safe foods that strengthen the health of your entire body. The Eczema Diet is incredibly nutritious, and as you or your child's eczema clears up, a wider variety of foods is reintroduced to the diet so you can enjoy most — if not all — foods and remain eczema-free. If you have severe allergies, continue to avoid your allergy foods until given clearance by your doctor.

Evidence-Based

Ten years later, my daughter is 12 years old and the
Eczema Diet program has changed a lot since I first
devised it. For the past decade, my eczema patients have
been giving me feedback about the program, which
has enabled me to refine the diet. One of the things
I love most about my job is reading research papers
on skin health. I'm often in my home office until well
past midnight, reading medical documents published
on eczema, even ones dating back to the 1800s — a
dangerous era to have eczema because doctors often
prescribed toxic heavy metals that occasionally caused
fatalities! In the late 1800s, some hospital-based doctors advocated dietary
changes, which were effective for treating eczema. By the mid-1900s,
topical steroids became popular and diet research slowed. However, in the
last 30 years, nutrition research into eczema has increased. This research
is referred to in the text and cited in the list of references. The information
we provide and the program we recommend are evidence-based. If you
have a baby with eczema, this research is still relevant to you because
you can use it to analyze your family diet when your baby starts eating
solids. Once the skin barrier function is restored, dust mites are no longer
a problem and you can resume normal activities, such as swimming and
playing with pets.

> The information we provide and the program we recommend are evidence-based.

Three-Stage Program

The Eczema Diet has three stages. In Stage 1, you are encouraged to
relieve your eczema symptoms by eating a restricted diet, limiting
yourself to eczema-healthy foods, and avoiding foods that aggravate your
symptoms. A series of guidelines is provided to help you change your
eating habits, with corresponding shopping lists, menu plans, and recipes.
Guidelines are also provided for using skin care products that can ease the
itch until the diet takes hold. This is the recovery stage of the program. In
Stage 2, you can begin to reintroduce some foods back into your diet as
your symptoms begin to disappear. Your diet now is less restricted, less
limited. In Stage 3, you consolidate your new eating habits, maintaining a
healthy acid-alkaline balance, a healthy fats ratio, and a healthy histamine
level, for example. Please keep in mind you will need to tailor this advice
to suit your individual case of eczema and other health concerns.

I know that right now, while you have eczema, it can be painful
and incredibly itchy. It can be heartbreaking to see your child or a close
friend suffering. Sometimes your toughest challenges call on you to find
new and more effective solutions, taking action on what really works for
you. I know the program will work for you, and I wish you well in your
endeavor to create beautiful, eczema-free skin.

Health and happiness,
Karen Fischer

Eczema at a Glance

Facts

Prevalence and Incidence Statistics

- 20% of the population of the Western world has eczema.
- In the United States, 15 million people have eczema.
- It's mostly babies and children who are suffering from eczema.
- One in five children suffers from eczema.
- Eczema sufferers in the United States spend up to $2,000 on eczema treatments each year.
- 36% of sufferers spend more than 10 minutes each day applying topical steroids and emollients.
- Despite the best medical care, the number of people with eczema continues to rise.

Genetic Risk Factors

Eczema is not contagious, so you can't catch it from someone if you touch their skin, breath, or blood. Most people with eczema inherited it from their parents.
- If you have one parent with eczema, you have a 20% risk of developing eczema yourself.
- If both parents suffer from eczema, hay fever, or asthma, your chances of developing eczema jump to between 50% and 80%.
- Your children inherit these same risk factors from you.

Dietary Changes

These eczema statistics and genetic risks may continue to rise and persist if we do not address the main factor that determines our genetic health: our diet.

- According to the Nutrition and Genomics Laboratory and the United States Department of Agriculture (USDA): "Food intake is the environmental factor to which we are all exposed permanently from conception to death. Therefore, dietary habits are the most important environmental factor modulating gene expression during one's life span."

- Although it is acceptable to use modern medicines to help you or your child gain temporary relief from eczema, a long-term solution involves dietary changes.

Eczema FAQs

During our years of using the Eczema Diet, we have been asked many questions. A core of frequently asked questions has emerged. As they say, there are no bad questions in medicine. Here are some short answers that are elaborated on in various places in the book.

Q. When will my skin begin to improve on this diet?

A. After strictly following the diet and supplement routine, your eczema should show signs of improvement within 2 weeks and should be mostly or completely clear by the eighth week. If you have suffered from eczema for many years, however, your body may take longer to detoxify and heal. Read the following FAQs to see what may be affecting your results.

Q. How do I know that I'm eating the right kind of food?

A. That's simple. Just follow the shopping guides and menu plans presented in this book. You need to eat plenty of alkalizing foods. If you eat too much acidic food, such as red meat, or too many carbohydrates, such as muffins, then you need to balance these meals with alkalizing vegetables at some point throughout the day (not necessarily within the same meal). You can do this by eating eczema-healthy vegetables and by drinking Tarzan Juice (page 207) or Healthy Skin Juice (page 206). Our eczema patients say these juices prevent their eczema from returning.

Q. Will I need to cleanse or detoxify my body in order to improve my chances of recovery?

A. Yes, the Eczema Diet features a gentle 3-day alkalizing cleanse accompanied by the consumption of a therapeutic broth. Adults can do the cleanse once a month if necessary, and make the therapeutic broth at least once every 14 days so you can flavor your meals, soups, and casseroles with this nutritious broth. Also ensure you are drinking plenty of filtered water. The programs for babies and children do not include a cleanse.

Q. How do I manage unforeseen food allergies and sensitivities?

A. One of our eczema patients (an 8-month-old baby) was following the diet along with his breastfeeding mother, and his eczema partially improved but did not completely heal as expected. The mother had a hunch to also take rice out of their diets — her son's eczema worsened after the introduction of baby rice cereal. Two weeks later, the eczema on her son's face completely cleared up. This was unexpected because rice allergy is very rare. In this patient's case, we substituted rice with barley, oats, and quinoa. Instead of rice bran oil, the mother used refined safflower oil (not antioxidant and not extra virgin) because this oil has a high smoking point, making it ideal for cooking. Instead of rice malt syrup, she used real maple syrup, golden syrup, or barley malt.

If you suspect you are reacting to a specific food item or food group, take it out of your diet for 2 weeks or more and see if your skin greatly improves. If you are taking these nutritious foods out of your diet, ensure you are taking an eczema supplement containing quercetin and vitamin C.

If you have no clue what foods or beverages may be affecting your skin, then varying the diet can help. For example, eliminate foods that have gluten (wheat, spelt, oats, rye, barley flour) for 2 weeks and then reintroduce these foods into your diet. If you react adversely, you are likely gluten intolerant.

Q. I've fallen off the sugar wagon. How can I manage the temptation to eat sweet pastries and candies?

A. Your eczema will not likely clear up if you continue eating sugary foods. Likewise, you need to avoid dairy foods. Don't despair. A number of eczema-safe sweeteners, such as rice malt syrup, and a number of cow's milk substitutes, such as rice milk and organic soy milk, are great substitutes.

continued...

Q. My 1-month-old son's eczema was improving, but then he woke up today in intense pain. What should I do?

A. Let us turn the questions back to you. Did anything in your child's routine change yesterday? For example, did you introduce any new foods? If you are breastfeeding, did you eat any new foods? Did you use teething gel to soothe his emerging teeth? Teething gel is rich in salicylates and is not eczema-safe. If you cannot pinpoint a cause of his pain, contact your physician for urgent care.

Q. I've been following the Eczema Diet program "religiously," but I'm still experiencing flare-ups. What do you advise?

A. Consider the cosmetics you are using. The wrong skin care products can cause flare-ups. Make sure you are using a skin cream, soap, and bath oil that don't irritate your skin. It is a process of trial and error to find the products that are right for you. Do this before you begin the Eczema Diet so you can tell if your skin cream is affecting your skin. Allergies to skin care products can also develop over time.

Q. My child is a fussy eater who won't eat the vegetables in this diet program. What can I do?

A. If your child is a fussy eater and won't eat the food or vegetables, then this program may be difficult to complete. The supplement regimen can help to partially heal the skin (especially the use of glycine), but supplements work best when combined with the food recommended in the Eczema Diet. Consult with your physician, pediatrician, or dietitian for strategies to help your child to enjoy eating vegetables.

Q. Does the Eczema Diet work for vegans and vegetarians?

A. Yes, but you will need to work harder and be more vigilant. If you are vegetarian or vegan, you may be eating products that are not eczema-safe. Tempeh, vegan patties, and other meat substitutes can contain additives. If you are vegan, you may be using an iron supplement that is plant- or herbal-based and is rich in salicylates, which, unfortunately, can cause flare-ups. Review the food lists provided in this book and note the foods that meet the double requirement of being eczema-safe and vegan compatible.

Q. Is it true that stress can affect skin health?

A. Work stress, relationship stress, emotional stress, and any kind of long-term stress can prevent your skin from clearing up. Stress can block enzyme reactions in the body and cause increased inflammation in susceptible individuals. If you are going through serious pain, grief, or loss, or have been through any kind of trauma, you may need to speak to a trusted psychotherapist, psychologist, or counselor who can help you work through emotional pain. This may take time, so be patient with and kind to yourself. Stress also triggers the production of acid in the body, so if you are stressed, you will need to eat plenty of alkaline vegetables.

Q. What can I eat when dining out?

A. Eating out is simple. Just order meals with skinless chicken, fish, lamb or beans with vegetables and rice. Ask for no sauces or dressings.

Q. How do I know if information on the Internet is credible?

A. Googling information can be risky and cause setbacks. Beware of combining the Eczema Diet with other programs that you may have read about online or received from a friend or relative. The Eczema Diet has been carefully designed for eczema, and each food has been researched and chosen for a specific reason — other foods may cause flare-ups.

Q. What is a diet diary?

A. A diet diary is a useful tool to help you record the meals you eat and rate how your skin looks at the end of the day. For example, a patient of mine kept experiencing occasional flare-ups, although her skin was improving on the Eczema Diet. I checked her diet diary and realized she was drinking herbal tea (which I had recommended for other skin conditions in my book *The Healthy Skin Diet*), so she was advised to stop drinking it. She was also eating candies whenever she felt tired. When she stopped consuming these, her eczema cleared up.

Diet Diary

Record your meals and rate your eczema.
Eczema rate: 1 is mild, 10 is unbearable. Do you see any connections between your diet and your eczema rate?

Meal	Monday	Tuesday	Wednesday
Breakfast			
Morning Snack			
Lunch			
Afternoon Snack			
Dinner			
Snack			
Rate your eczema:	___/10	___/10	___/10

Thursday	Friday	Saturday	Sunday
___/10	___/10	___/10	___/10

Part 1

Getting to Know Eczema

Chapter 1
Skin Basics

∙∙∙∙∙∙∙∙∙∙∙∙∙∙∙∙∙∙∙∙∙∙∙∙∙∙∙∙∙∙∙∙∙∙∙∙∙

Testimonial

Georgia's skin condition has really started clearing up over the past 4 to 5 weeks. Georgia (Gigi) woke up a couple of days ago and said, "Mom, I don't have eczema anymore!" She was so excited. She still has lots of scar tissue on her feet and on the backs of her knees that I hope in time will fade, but all the redness, inflammation, and soreness have gone. You are a true blessing, Karen. I'm so excited! Life for us have never been better and I can thank you for most of that! Ever since Gigi was 8 months old, I have tried every doctor, dermatologist, naturopath, and dietitian in our community, but no one has explained eczema to me like you have. Your book is a bible and should have a place in everybody's home.

Amanda Essex

How the Skin Works

Your skin is not only something you hope (and pray) looks good as you step through your front door each day. Like your heart and lungs, your skin is a vital organ that keeps you alive. Your skin is a barrier and a filter between the outside world and your insides — which is why the outermost layer of skin, the stratum corneum, is known as the skin barrier. A normal skin barrier is thick, and the outermost layers of dead skin cells flake off in a barely detectable manner as the outermost binders snap and release the unwanted cells. New skin cells form at the

Functions of the Skin

- Protects your body from excessive water loss so you don't die from dehydration.
- Helps to regulate your body temperature so you don't "cook" your internal organs.
- Protects you from invading microbes, such as dust mites and bacteria.

bottom of the epidermis, and when they are ready, they move toward the stratum corneum. In normal, healthy skin, this trip takes about 4 weeks.

Q. What goes wrong with the skin when you have eczema?

A. First, the skin barrier does not function normally and becomes too thin, which results in "leaky skin." Whatever comes in contact with the skin barrier tends to soak into the deeper layers of the skin. The skin barrier becomes abnormally dry and sensitive as moisturizing oils are carried away. This dry skin becomes excessively itchy and a rash results. Eczema is sometimes called "the itch that rashes."

Skin Anatomy

New skin cells form at the bottom of the epidermis, and when they're ready, they move towards the stratum corneum. In normal, healthy skin this trip takes about 4 weeks.

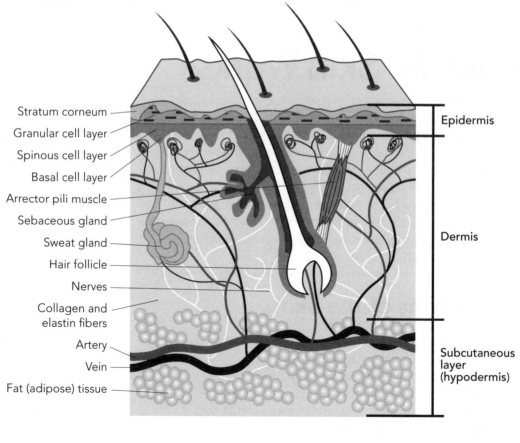

Stratum corneum
Granular cell layer
Spinous cell layer
Basal cell layer
Arrector pili muscle
Sebaceous gland
Sweat gland
Hair follicle
Nerves
Collagen and elastin fibers
Artery
Vein
Fat (adipose) tissue

Epidermis

Dermis

Subcutaneous layer (hypodermis)

Q. How do I know if I have eczema?

A. Eczema is generally diagnosed using well-established criteria. You must have itchy skin, plus three or more of the following symptoms:

- Itchiness in the skin creases and folds behind the knees and in the elbows, in the front of the ankles, and around the neck (children under 4 years old may also have it on their cheeks)
- Dry skin
- Visible eczema rash affecting the outer limbs, cheeks, or forehead
- Symptoms appearing within 2 years of birth (not always an indication, but very common)
- Family history of asthma, hay fever, or (if under 4 years old) atopic disease in a first-degree relative

Know Your Lingo

Atopic: describes an allergy-prone individual and includes eczema, asthma, and hay fever.
Dermatitis: refers to any generalized inflammation of the skin.
Eczema: is derived from a Greek word meaning "to boil out." Eczema also refers to dermatitis, unless otherwise stated.

Brick Wall Model

A useful way to describe the basic structural changes the skin goes through when you have eczema is demonstrated in the "brick wall" model of the skin, which was created by Professor Michael Cork and colleagues at the University of Sheffield in the United Kingdom. In this model, skin cells are likened to bricks held together by iron rods (binders called corneodesmosomes) and mortar (lipids, which are fats).

When you have eczema, the skin barrier is usually thinner than normal, so its protective capacity is compromised. The binders that hold the skin cells together in the deeper layers of the skin snap too early, causing premature flaking of the skin. The fatty lipids in between your skin cells have cracks that appear throughout the skin barrier.

Irritants, including soaps and detergents, enhance the snapping-off process of the binders. The skin cells break down prematurely and deeper cracks appear in the skin. As the skin barrier breaks down, the cracks allow allergens, such as dust mites and bacteria, to enter the skin. This contributes to flare-ups and can lead to infections and immune responses, including allergic reactions.

Brick Wall Model of the Skin Barrier

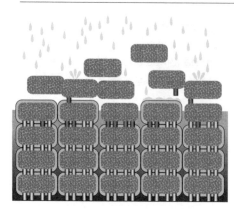
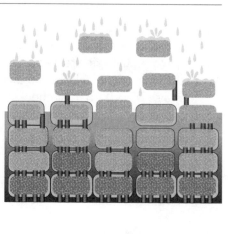
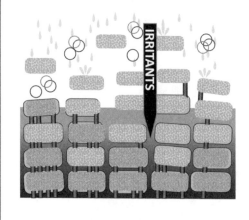
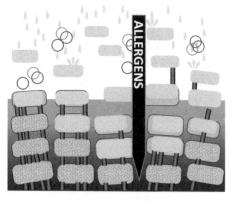

(Adapted with permission from Cork and Hunter)

Acid Mantle

With the exception of newborn babies (who have a skin pH that is close to neutral), healthy skin has an acidic pH of approximately 5.5. This is known as the "acid mantle." The acid mantle protects the skin from harmful microbes, decreases the colonization of freeloading pathogenic bacteria and fungi, and promotes the adhesion to the skin of beneficial (non-pathogenic) bacteria. Research shows that eczema sufferers can have skin that is not acidic enough, making the skin barrier less protective and practically defenseless against microbes, such as dust mites and *Staphylococcus aureus*.

Infected Eczema

Having eczema can sometimes make you feel as if you are sitting on top of an ant's nest. Sometimes you just end up scratching even though you know you shouldn't. Scratching causes broken skin and an increased risk of bacterial, viral, and fungal skin infections, impetigo, and cold sores (herpes simplex virus type 1). All are good reasons to avoid scratching your skin. Infections can also delay the healing of eczema, so it is important to identify and treat infections early.

How do you know if your skin has become infected? It is sometimes difficult to spot an infection, but if your eczema suddenly worsens and does not respond to topical treatments, you should suspect an infection and see your doctor immediately. Not all signs and symptoms of infected eczema will be present at one time.

Symptoms of Infected Eczema

- Hot and sore skin that is red and angry
- Weepy/yellowish crust
- Pus
- Folliculitis (small inflamed red spots, especially around hair follicles)
- Tender, swollen glands in the neck, groin, or armpits
- Signs of candida/fungal infection: red, itchy, and sore skin and possibly tiny yellow pustules; white patches on the skin
- Impetigo
- Cold sores (herpes simplex virus type 1)
- Signs of eczema herpeticum: small blisters containing clear fluid or yellow pus, which break open and ulcerate; high temperature; general unwell feeling

Infection Care

If you suspect you have an infection, see a doctor or visit your local hospital emergency room. Your doctor can do a fast and painless swab test to help identify the cause of the infection. Swabs help to identify which prescription would be most effective at eradicating the infection before it spreads and becomes dangerous. For example, the test may reveal the skin is infected with the bacteria *Staphylococcus aureus* or *Streptococcus*, and these would require a vastly different treatment to a *Candida albicans* fungal infection. By quickly treating your skin with the most appropriate medication, the infection should rapidly clear up.

Guidelines for Preventing Eczema Infections

Even when you take the best care of your skin, it's not always possible to prevent eczema from becoming infected. However, you can reduce the risk of skin infections by following these guidelines.

1. Follow the Eczema Diet. This diet boosts the immune system and promotes healthy skin barrier function so it can reduce the risk of infection.
2. Avoid scratching itchy skin.
3. Minimize the itch by consuming alkalizing foods and drinks.
4. Do not share towels and facecloths with other family members, especially if they have an infection, such as a cold sore.
5. Protect the skin's barrier and reduce dryness and cracking with the daily use of moisturizing creams and bath oils.
6. Avoid soaps and dehydrating environments (such as air-conditioning and electric heating) that dry out the skin and increase the risk of skin cracking.
7. Only use skin care products that contain preservatives (preservatives prevent bacterial growth in a skin care product).
8. Wash your hands frequently using a gentle hand soap (especially before applying emollients to your eczema).
9. Avoid using old or out-of-date skin care products.
10. Avoid using old or out-of-date makeup.

Did You Know?

Dietary Modification

American researchers claim that our dietary habits are the most important environmental factor modulating gene expression. According to German researchers, essential fatty acids in the diet can modify gene expression, T-cell function, cell membrane fluidity, and cell signaling. In experimental studies, dietary carotenoids have been shown to modulate gene activity to protect against inflammatory damage and tumor growth. In one of the largest gene-diet interaction studies ever conducted, involving the analysis of more than 27,000 people from five ethnic groups (European, South Asian, Chinese, Latin American, and Arab), the effect of diet on genetic health was confirmed yet again. Researchers reported that a healthy diet rich in raw vegetables and fruit modified the gene variants located on chromosome 9p21, which is the strongest marker for heart disease. A healthy diet significantly weakened this gene's damaging effects.

Nature or Nurture?

Eczema is a unique skin disease with many associated causal factors. Although no single one of these factors categorically causes eczema, genetics and diet play central roles.

Genetic Defects

Eczema is not contagious, so you can't catch it from someone if you touch their skin, breath, or blood. If you have eczema, chances are that you inherited it from your parents. According to research studies, eczema is regulated by approximately four or five major genes. Some affect the immune system, while others weaken the skin barrier. All genes come in pairs, and some eczema sufferers can have one or two defective copies of the filaggrin genes (the protein that binds keratin fibers in the epithelial cells in human tissue). Approximately 10% of the British population has a single defective copy, which causes them to suffer from dry, flaking skin.

Primitive Diet

Your diet affects your genetic health in a variety of ways. In the *American Journal of Clinical Nutrition*, Professor Loren Cordain claims that we have not kept pace biologically with the evolution of the Western diet — from primitive hunting and gathering to domestic crop growing and animal husbandry. Human genetics may be in the process of adapting to these food practices, but in the meantime, the domestic Western diet, high in refined sugar and white flour, poses many dietary challenges for eczema patients:

- Fewer micronutrients are present in the typical Western diet. Processed foods often contain sugar and white flour, which are low in vitamins and minerals.
- Glycemic load has increased. Glycemic load is a measure of our blood glucose and insulin levels immediately after eating a specific food. Processed Western foods usually have a higher glycemic load, which can result in diabetes, heart disease, and eczema.

> Eczema is not contagious, so you can't catch it from someone if you touch their skin, breath, or blood. If you have eczema, chances are that you inherited it from your parents.

Did You Know?

....

Nutrient
Deficiency

Deficiency in just
a single nutrient
can trigger a
genetic defect
that leads to the
onset of eczema.
Your health-care
provider may ask
to conduct blood,
hair, and urine tests
to determine if
you are deficient
in any nutrient and
then recommend
specific foods and
supplements to help
you meet this need.

- Fat ratios have increased. The National Institutes of Health report that the ratio for omega-6 and omega-3 essential fatty acids was 1:1 in the primitive diet, but in our current diet, the ratio is 15:1 to 16:1. The result is an increased risk of heart disease and diabetes.

- Acid-alkaline balance has been altered. Foods in the Western diet are predominantly acidic and can affect the skin's acid mantle, as well as cause low-grade metabolic acidosis that worsens with age.

- Sodium-potassium ratio has also altered. There has been a 400% increase in salt ingestion, while potassium-rich fruit and vegetable consumption has plummeted.

- Fiber content has decreased. Fiber is essential for the digestion and absorption of nutrients. Sugars, vegetable oils, alcohol, and dairy products are devoid of fiber, and refined grains contain much less fiber than whole grains.

Chapter 2
Six-Step Anti-Eczema Program

Testimonials

My 4-year-old daughter, who is about to start kindergarten, has been taken off preservatives and artificial colors and has been taking her supplements for her severe eczema and is looking like a million dollars. What a difference in just 6 weeks. After 4 years of battling her eczema (not sleeping, not eating, extreme fatigue, and hospitalization with infected skin), I am now in control, more than ever. The doctors told me it was all about maintaining her comfort. The Eczema Diet maintenance program is sooooo much better than the many, many tubes of cortisone cream that I used to use.

Meaghan Ottewill

The Eczema Diet is a holistic health program that incorporates both the avoidance of offending substances and the addition of eczema-healthy foods and nutrients to boost the health of your liver, blood, and gastrointestinal tract — and restore skin health. Clinical research on eczema, conducted in university laboratories and private clinics by scientists, doctors, and professors around the world during the past 60 years, has shown us how diet is linked to skin health and the onset of eczema. Here are six techniques to empower you in your efforts to conquer eczema.

> Clinical research has shown us how diet is linked to skin health and the onset of eczema.

How the Eczema Diet Works

The Eczema Diet is designed to:

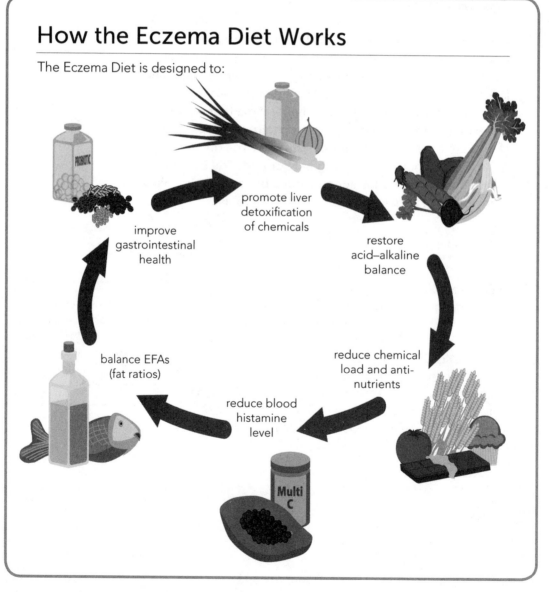

improve gastrointestinal health

promote liver detoxification of chemicals

restore acid–alkaline balance

reduce chemical load and anti-nutrients

reduce blood histamine level

balance EFAs (fat ratios)

Reduce Your Chemical Load

During the past 200 years, food manufacturers have introduced highly processed foods containing artificial colors, preservatives, sweeteners, and flavor enhancers. However, our biological makeup has not had enough time to become accustomed to this barrage of artificial additives. According to some authorities, there were more than 1,000 products in 2009 containing problematic food colorings that can worsen eczema symptoms and cause a range of side effects. Population studies confirm that acne and eczema are rare in traditional cultures where processed foods are not a regular part of the diet. Eating little or no food with additives will help control your eczema, but avoiding these foods is not easy. Not all ingredients are listed on food labels.

Additives to Avoid

Various agencies, such as the Federal Drug Administration in the United States and Health Canada, assign numbers to these additives for ease of identification. For example, the natural coloring annatto is numbered 160b. Check with these agencies for additional information on the identification and safety of additives.

Additive	Food Source
Flavor enhancers: glutamates, monosodium glutamate (MSG)	Flavored noodles, flavored crackers, chips, stock cubes, gravies, fast foods, and Chinese foods MSG include tomatoes, soy sauce, broccoli, mushrooms, spinach, grapes, plums, deli meats, miso, tempeh, wine, rum, sherry, brandy, and liqueur
Artificial colorings	Confectionery, candy, jelly, breakfast cereals, glacé cherries, salmon feed, hot dogs, soda, flavored mineral water, chocolate, potato chips, corn chips, toppings, ice cream, ice pops (Ice pops), fruit drinks, cordials, flavored milks, meat pies, cupcakes, cakes, liqueur, yogurt, and dairy snacks
Natural coloring	Many yogurts, butter, fish sticks, custard, and commercial desserts
Preservatives: sorbates, benzoates, sulfites, nitrates, nitrites, propionates	Some processed fruits and vegetables, wine, beer, most sodas, diet drinks, cordials, juices, processed meats, sausages, dried fruit, and deli meats; number 282 is found in some breads, buns, and wraps
Antioxidant preservatives	Oils, margarines, french fries, fried snack foods, fast foods
Artificial sweeteners: aspartame, saccharin, sucralose	NutraSweet, Equal, Sweet'N Low, diet and "sugar-free" products, diet sodas, "zero" sodas, cakes, cookies, sweet pies, muffins, and ice cream

(Adapted from http://fedup.com.au/ McCann, D. et al. Food additives and hyperactive behaviour in 3-year-old and 8/9-year-old children in the community: a randomised, double-blinded, placebo-controlled trial. The Lancet. 370:1560–67; Dengate S. Food Intolerance Network Fact Sheet).

Chemical Sensitivities

How do you know if you have a sensitivity to a specific chemical? Chemical sensitivity is an adverse reaction that can occur within 3 hours or up to several days after coming into contact with the offending chemical. Symptoms are varied. They can be mild to severe, depending on the individual, and include skin rashes, migraines, headaches, depression, irritability, unfocused behavior, hyperactivity, flu-like symptoms, and a worsening of eczema symptoms. In severe cases, some sensitivities can trigger physical pain and strong feelings of anger, aggression, and even suicidal thoughts. Some of these chemicals are considered to be natural, such as salicylates, and others are artificial, such as nitrites and nitrates.

Salicylates

Ingesting salicylate-rich foods can cause a worsening of eczema symptoms. Salicylates are chemicals found naturally in many fruits and vegetables, herbs, nuts, teas, coffee, wine, beer, and spices. Salicylates are also used in many skin creams and perfumes. According to research from the Royal Prince Alfred Hospital Allergy Unit in Sydney, Australia, salicylate sensitivity is the most common chemical sensitivity in eczema sufferers. A high dose of salicylates (especially if taking aspirin, which contains salicylates) can cause temporary damage to the stomach lining, especially in children and sensitive individuals.

Salicylates are often touted as an eczema sufferer's worst enemy, but are they to be permanently avoided? Maybe not. Salicylates are often found in the most nutritious foods, such as dark green leafy vegetables and blueberries, so you want to do all you can to prevent or decrease your salicylate sensitivity. Here is the key: your liver is designed to detoxify salicylates and other chemicals so they can be safely removed from the body. In order for this to occur, your diet (or the maternal diet if your eczema-prone baby is being breastfed) needs to supply all the nutrients the liver requires for salicylate detoxification. These nutrients are glycine, vitamin B6, and magnesium.

Nitrates

Nitrates are chemicals used to preserve meats, chiefly bacon, sausages, and ham. Nitrates are also found in the nettings used to wrap deli meats and in tobacco smoke. In the 1970s, it was discovered that harmful nitrosamines form during the cooking of nitrate-containing meats, and these can cause cancer and liver damage. Recent research has shown that eczema sufferers are sensitive to nitrates. Nitrate consumption aggravated eczema symptoms in 43% of the eczema patients being studied.

Your diet can help to reduce the damaging effects of nitrates. According to laboratory studies, the antioxidants quercetin, vitamin C, and vitamin E help to reverse the liver damage caused by nitrate consumption.

Food Coloring

If you have ever eaten food at a children's party, chances are you have ingested dozens of artificial food colorings that are known to exacerbate eczema. These food colorings are added to brightly colored party food. Regular breakfast cereals, yogurt, and margarines also contain food colorings that can trigger a range of adverse reactions, including eczema symptoms.

The food coloring known as tartrazine (102), one of several yellow food colorings, has been shown to adversely impact eczema symptoms in 40% of eczema sufferers. It can also trigger asthma attacks, runny nose, purplish skin bruising, and, in severe cases, anaphylactic shock.

How can eating a yellow candy cause such problems? Tartrazine stimulates the production of pro-inflammatory leukotrienes. A team of researchers at Southampton University in the United Kingdom also found that artificial colorings can hamper a child's intelligence by up to five IQ points and cause behavioral problems, such as inattention and hyperactivity.

Did You Know?

Annatto (160b)

Artificial colorings are not the only additives eczema sufferers should avoid. There is also a natural food coloring that is problematic. Most children consume it on a daily basis. Annatto, used to color many brands of butter, yogurt, and fish sticks, to name a few sources, has been reported to cause eczema flare-ups in sensitive individuals. Adverse reactions to annatto include obsessive head banging, irritable bowel syndrome, headaches, and learning difficulties. Surprisingly, some children may obsessively favor yellow: for example, they only want yellow food/pencils/clothes — but this obsession ceases when annatto is removed from the diet. In Europe, annatto has been banned from use in foods, and a safe alternative, beta-carotene (160a), is used instead.

Sulfites

Sulfites, such as sulfur dioxide, are food preservatives commonly used to preserve wines, deli meats, dried fruits, and dried vegetables, to name a few processed foods. Sulfites destroy vitamin B_1 and folate in foods. They are considered to be an "anti-nutrient." Although dried fruits might be touted as a healthy snack for children, studies have shown that one dried apricot can contain 16 mg of sulfur dioxide, which can aggravate eczema symptoms in susceptible individuals and cause a range of adverse reactions, such as diarrhea, unfocused behavior, hyperactivity, and smelly gas. It could also trigger an asthma attack in susceptible individuals.

If you have ever experienced facial flushing after drinking a glass of red wine or consuming vinegar, you may be sensitive to sulfites. Highly sensitive people may react to sulfur-rich garlic and onions.

Q. What is sulfur sensitivity?

A. Sulfur is an essential element for making proteins in body cells, hair, and nails. The sulfur in vegetables can assist the liver in its role of cleansing the body of toxins, which is why vegetables feature heavily in the Eczema Diet. Although most people can eat sulfur-containing foods with no problems, a few are highly sensitive to them, particularly garlic and onions (leeks and green onions are part of the onion family). Sulfur-rich foods include Brussels sprouts, cauliflower, asparagus, and eggs. If you are highly sensitive to sulfur, you may not be able to tolerate alpha-lipoic acid, although the dosages recommended in the supplement section (page 94) are at a lower dosage and should be well tolerated.

Monosodium Glutamate

Monosodium glutamate (MSG) is a flavor enhancer that is both natural (present in tomato) and artificially produced (added to potato chips). One study found that 35% of eczema sufferers have adverse reactions to dietary MSG. MSG may increase the risk of premature wrinkles because it reduces stores of glutathione, an anti-aging antioxidant enzyme needed for the liver detoxification of chemicals. In animal studies, MSG ingestion produced liver inflammation, which significantly increases the size of the liver and promotes liver damage.

Q. Can modifying your diet now make up for previous dietary sins?

A. Clinical studies show MSG-induced liver damage can be reversed with antioxidant supplementation. Consuming soy sauce, fermented soybeans, chocolate, cheese, coffee, and yogurt causes a worsening of eczema symptoms, according to a Japanese study published in the *Journal of Dermatology*. After the avoidance of these foods for 3 months, all the participating eczema sufferers had reduced eczema symptoms.

Guidelines for Reducing Your Chemical Load

- Avoid consuming artificial additives in your diet.
- Eat organic foods grown without chemical fertilizers and pesticides.
- Wash fruits and vegetables in water to remove pesticides, soaking them for several minutes.
- Use a soft scrubbing brush on hardy fruits and vegetables, and peel the skin when possible.
- Avoid natural MSG sources, such as soy sauce, tomatoes, and grapes, as well as other flavor enhancers.
- Avoid sulfite-rich foods and drinks, including sulphite-treated dried fruits and alcoholic beverages.
- Greatly reduce salicylate intake (some healthy salicylate foods are essential in the diet, specifically carrots, sweet potato, and beets, which supply carotenoids for skin protection).
- Avoid aspirin and baby teething gels because they are rich in salicylates.
- If you have been prescribed aspirin for heart disease, do not stop taking aspirin, but talk to your doctor about your options.
- Avoid nitrate-containing meats because they increase cancer risk and eczema symptoms.
- Avoid the natural color annatto (160b).
- Supplement with the antioxidants vitamin C, vitamin E, and alpha-lipoic acid.
- Supplement with the correct doses of glycine, magnesium, and vitamin B6. (Do not take glycine if you are on blood-thinning medications, such as aspirin.)

Reduce Your Blood Histamine Levels

An allergy is an abnormal immune response triggered by a normally harmless substance that results in a release of histamines into the blood. In eczema sufferers, allergic reactions can make eczema symptoms worse, including coughing, sneezing, wheezing, and, in severe instances, anaphylactic shock, a life-threatening swelling of the tongue or throat. Allergic reactions can be measured: allergy sufferers have raised levels of immunoglobulin E (IgE), the antibody found in your blood and tissues that mediates allergy.

Allergy Tests

There are different kinds of allergy tests, including the skin-prick test, the measuring of serum-specific IgE, and — for children under the age of 3 — a skin application food test. IgE-dependent food-allergic reactions cause a sharp rise in the blood histamine level and histamine toxicity occurs, which causes the negative symptoms you experience when you are having an allergic reaction.

Common Food Allergies Associated with Eczema

Food	Percentage of eczema patients with allergy
Eggs (chicken)	71%
Peanuts	65%
Dairy products, including cow's milk	38%
Tree nuts	34%
Sesame seeds	18%
Wheat	13%
Soy	4%

Dairy Allergy and Lactose Intolerance

Cow's milk proteins, casein and whey, can cause damage to the lining of the gastrointestinal tract. Research shows the consumption of cow's milk causes gastrointestinal bleeding in 50% of American infants who present with iron deficiency (frequent milk consumption can also cause iron-deficiency anemia). When the gut lining is damaged from eating dairy products, tiny holes allow larger food particles to enter the body and allergic reactions can result. Naturopaths often refer to this as leaky gut syndrome, but the medical term is increased intestinal permeability.

Lactose is the sugar that is found naturally in milk and dairy products like yogurt, butter, and cheese. In order for your body to break down lactose, you require the enzyme lactase in your digestive tract. If you are sensitive to dairy products, it is likely that your body does not adequately produce this enzyme. Lactose intolerance can cause diarrhea, gas, cramps, and bloating. More than 40% of eczema sufferers are sensitive to lactose and they experience an increase of eczema symptoms when they consume lactose.

Allergic March

During the past 20 years, researchers have found that food allergies in 40% of infants and young children with moderate to severe eczema resolve in early childhood. There is, however, an increased risk of atopic march, also known as the allergic march. Atopic march means that the allergic response changes as the child grows older. For example, a child under the age of 3 with eczema and allergies grows out of the allergies, but more serious symptoms of asthma — wheezing and difficulty breathing — develop. In the adolescent years, when asthma begins to subside, hay fever symptoms occur. Later in life, at about the age of 40, just as allergic rhinitis is settling down, asthma and eczema return. Research shows that antihistamine drugs, which are often prescribed to eczema sufferers, fail to prevent the atopic march, but diet can alleviate symptoms and reduce the risk.

Reduce Histamines

Your body not only makes histamine in response to an allergic reaction, your food also supplies histamines and other amines. According to several research papers, eczema sufferers have elevated histamine levels in the blood, combined with a reduced capacity to detoxify these histamines. When they eat amine-rich foods, 36% of eczema sufferers experience a worsening of eczema symptoms.

Allergy Symptoms Questionnaire

Allergy tests are useful, but keep in mind they only identify a limited number of possible food allergies, and even if you have been tested for allergies, you may still be exposing yourself to foods you are sensitive to. Complete this questionnaire to see if you have food or environmental allergy symptoms. Use a checkmark to highlight the answer that best suits your experience (yes = weekly or daily; sometimes = monthly or occasionally; no = never or rarely; unsure = not known).

ALLERGY SYMPTOM	Yes	Sometimes	No	Unsure
Do you have any of the following?				
1. Nasal symptoms				
Itchy nose				
Nasal drip				
Blocked or stuffy nose				
Sneezing				
Wheezing				
Crease at the end of the nose from frequent rubbing/itching/wiping of drips				
2. Skin symptoms				
Hives				
Skin rash				
Itchy skin				
Eczema				
Facial flushing				
Rosacea				
Acne				
Foul or abnormal body odor				
Excessive perspiration				
Swelling (lips, tongue, eyes, throat)				
3. Eye symptoms				
Dark rings under the eyes (allergic shiners)				
Puffy eyes				
Itchy eyes				
Conjunctivitis				
Eye pain				
Temporary blurred vision				
4. Gastrointestinal symptoms				
Diarrhea				
Constipation				

ALLERGY SYMPTOM	Yes	Sometimes	No	Unsure
Colic				
Excessive or smelly gas				
Indigestion				
Gastrointestinal bleeding				
Nausea				
Stomach or abdominal cramps/pains				
Vomiting				
Bad breath				
Loss of appetite				
Acid reflux				
5. Headache symptoms				
Headaches/migraines				
6. Blood pressure symptoms				
Low blood pressure				
High blood pressure				
Heart palpitations				
Quickened pulse after consuming a particular food or being exposed to an allergen				
7. Musculoskeletal symptoms				
Muscle aches and pains				
Joint pain				
Muscle weakness				
8. Behavioral symptoms				
Hyperactivity (attention deficit disorder, ADD; attention deficit/hyperactivity disorder, ADHD)				
Anxiety				
Temporary confusion				
Intense cravings (often for the food you are allergic to)				
Mood changes after eating				
Sleep problems (insomnia or the excessive need for sleep)				

Score: If you experience three or more of these allergy symptoms, you could have undiagnosed allergies or food/chemical/environmental sensitivities. Other health factors may also be involved. If you have any concerns, speak to your doctor for a formal diagnosis. In the meantime, keep a diet diary to help you identify what you ate preceding an attack (for a sample diet diary, see page 16).

Symptoms of histamine toxicity are the same as the symptoms of an allergic reaction: a runny nose or nasal obstruction can be the first sign. Other symptoms include skin rash, a worsening of eczema symptoms, headaches, diarrhea, stomach ache, colic, flatulence, sneezing, asthma, and facial flushing. Histamine toxicity occurs when the blood histamine level elevates beyond what the liver is capable of detoxifying. The health of your liver is an important part of managing allergic reactions and eczema.

Antihistamine Treatments

Medications that are often prescribed to eczema sufferers do not improve DAO activity. These antihistamine drugs suppress the liver's ability to detoxify histamines. In other words, these drugs mask the symptoms when an allergic reaction occurs, but they fail to treat the cause.

Although antihistamine drugs can be useful in emergencies, there is a healthy alternative: papaya. According to research published in the *American Journal of Clinical Nutrition,* vitamin C and vitamin B6 increase DAO activity and break down histamine, and both vitamins can be found in papaya.

Laboratory experiments also show that the flavonoid quercetin, which is present in onions and is available as a supplement, also breaks down histamine.

Reduce Anti-Nutrients

Although it is impossible to totally eliminate anti-nutrients from your diet, high intakes of anti-nutrients can be problematic for eczema sufferers because they interfere with the absorption of skin-repairing minerals.

There are two main ways anti-nutrients lower nutrients in the body. First, anti-nutrients can require a range of vitamins and minerals in order for the body to digest and detoxify them, and they rob these nutrients from your body in the process. For example, packaged foods rich in sugar and white flour are low in nutrients, so although they satisfy your hunger, they do not supply the nutrients your body needs for healthy skin — plus they rob some of your body's stores of vitamins and minerals during digestion and detoxification (which means fewer nutrients for skin repair and maintenance).

Second, anti-nutrients can bind to nutrients in a way that stops your body from being able to use them. For example, avidin, a protein in raw egg whites, is an anti-nutrient because it binds to biotin and frequent consumption causes a deficiency. Dermatitis is the first symptom to follow. Phytic acid is another anti-nutrient, which binds to the minerals calcium, iron, zinc, and copper. Most types of grains and legumes, although an important source of dietary fiber to cleanse the bowel of toxins and cancer-causing substances, contain phytic acid. It is for this reason that you should soak grains, legumes, and nuts. This is easy to do. See "Soaking Grains" (page 76) and "Guidelines for Cooking Legumes" (page 82).

Supply Antihistamine Nutrients

The Eczema Diet ensures you are consuming the key antihistamine nutrients vitamin C, vitamin B6, and quercetin. Although these are provided in foods, such as papaya, mung bean sprouts, Brussels sprouts, and green onions, you need to supplement these food sources to help minimize allergic reactions and prevent histamine toxicity. Refer to Part 3, Eczema Supplements.

Guidelines for Reducing Allergies and Histamines

Eczema sufferers with allergies, especially those with life-threatening anaphylactic reactions, should continue to avoid the offending foods until given clearance by their doctor.

- If you experience serious swelling in your mouth or throat, stop eating and go to a hospital for emergency care because you may be having an anaphylactic reaction.
- Avoid all dairy products while you have eczema, but maintain healthy calcium levels by eating calcium-rich foods and taking calcium supplements if needed.
- Take natural antihistamines (vitamin C, vitamin B6, and quercetin) on a daily basis to reduce the risk of histamine toxicity and allergic reactions.
- Eat papaya and Brussels sprouts, because they are rich in vitamin C.

Improve Your Gastrointestinal Health

The Eczema Diet is designed to be gentle on your gastrointestinal tract. Foods and drinks that can cause intestinal permeability are taken out of the diet and a probiotic supplement can be taken if desired. Once your gastrointestinal health has strengthened, you can slowly reintroduce a wider range of foods into your diet. If you find you are still sensitive to a particular food, you should avoid it for another 2 months and then try eating it again if desired. When reintroducing these foods, introduce one new food every 3 days so you can clearly identify problematic foods.

Gut Barrier

Like your skin barrier, your gastrointestinal tract is your gut barrier — a vital part of your body's defense system against food-borne bacteria, toxins, and allergens. According to Italian researchers, children with eczema often have abnormalities in the gastrointestinal tract, including increased intestinal permeability. A clinical trial revealed 44% of children with atopic eczema have gastrointestinal symptoms after ingesting food compared with 22% of children without eczema. The most common gastrointestinal symptoms in children with eczema are diarrhea, regurgitation, and vomiting. These gastrointestinal symptoms were, in most cases, reported to have been present before the appearance of eczema. This research suggests that poor gastrointestinal health can contribute to the onset of eczema.

Like a vicious cycle, intestinal permeability can also occur after you have had an allergic response to food. When a food allergy triggers histamine to be released from mast cells, inflammation and increased vascular permeability occurs. Research shows that the intestinal mucosal defect in eczema sufferers can also exist in eczema patients who don't have food allergies.

Intestinal Permeability

Your diet plays a major role in your gastrointestinal health. What happens when you ignore your diet and fail to protect the gut lining from damage? Intestinal permeability creates a heavy workload for the liver, which can lead to damaged liver cells (hepatocytes) and increased free radicals in the bile. The liver is designed to detoxify substances, such as alcohol, and it makes bile to transport toxins to the colon for removal via the feces. Your diet directly affects how adequately your body eliminates toxin-loaded bile from the colon. The liver produces up to 4 cups (1 L) of bile salts every day, and to do this, it needs lecithin from your diet. Your body also needs plenty of dietary fiber to push chemical-loaded bile through the colon and to cleanse the colon of toxic substances, microbes, and carcinogens (substances that can cause cancer).

Causes of Intestinal Permeability

- Alcohol consumption (also damages stomach lining)
- Cow's milk consumption can cause gastrointestinal bleeding in infants
- Allergic reactions (releases histamine)
- Eating hot chile peppers frequently can damage the stomach lining
- Toxic bile
- Fungal infestation (e.g., candidiasis or parasite infestation)
- Wheat consumption, especially gluten protein
- Artificial additives consumption (e.g., preservatives)
- Excess salicylate consumption
- Aspirin or other non-steroidal anti-inflammatory drugs (NSAIDs)

Candida albicans Infestation

Another gastrointestinal problem common in eczema sufferers is fungal infestation. Research shows that 70% of patients with atopic eczema have *Candida albicans* overgrowth in the gastrointestinal tract. Furthermore, 69% of infants with seborrheic eczema, which affects the scalp, are infected with *Candida albicans* overgrowth at one or more external areas of the skin (including the inside of the mouth). Researchers suggest this may be linked to the use of topical steroid creams (which is another reason why cortisone creams should only be used in the short term, if at all). Overgrowth of pathogenic fungus, particularly *Malassezia* and candida, can trigger skin inflammation and increase the incidence of atopic eczema. When you have candida overgrowth, eczema symptoms cannot improve, even with a healthy diet, so it is essential to treat the fungal problem.

> **Did You Know?**
> ....
> **Alcohol-Induced Damage**
> In experimental studies, the antioxidant quercetin has been shown to protect the stomach lining from alcohol-induced damage, if taken during or prior to exposure.

> **Did You Know?**
> ....
> **Brewer's Yeast**
> Approximately 31% of eczema sufferers experience a worsening of eczema symptoms after consuming brewer's yeast. Brewer's yeast is a fungal micro-organism used to ferment carbohydrates in beer. It is available as a nutrition supplement.

Candida albicans Questionnaire

Complete this questionnaire to see if you have symptoms of *Candida albicans*. Use a checkmark to highlight the answer that best describes the frequency of that symptom or collection of symptoms (yes = weekly or daily; sometimes = monthly or occasionally; no = never or rarely; unsure = not known).

ALLERGY SYMPTOM	Yes	Sometimes	No	Unsure
Do you have any of the following?				
1. Visible signs of fungal infection on the skin				
Red, itchy skin				
Tiny yellow pustules				
White patches on the skin that show improvement with antifungal treatment				
Oral signs of candidiasis/yeast infection, which may look like white furry patches inside the mouth				
Did you have oral thrush as a baby or did your mother have a vaginal thrush infection during pregnancy or birth?				
2. Signs of thrush				
Genital itching/burning				
White or chalky discharge or appearance				
Stinging while urinating				
Other				
Do you take the birth control pill or undergo hormone replacement therapy?				
Have you used steroids/cortisone topically or orally for more than a month?				
Have you required several courses of antibiotics in the last year?				
Do you crave carbohydrates, such as sugar, sodas, juice, fruit, bread, or alcohol?				
Do you need caffeine (coffee, tea, soda, chocolate) each day to "wake up" or feel good?				
Do you experience stomach bloating after eating?				
Have you experienced changes in bowel movements or unpleasant gas?				
Have you been diagnosed with inflammatory bowel disease?				

Are you sensitive to perfume, perfumed products, household cleaners, and/or cigarette smoke?				
Are you sensitive to chemicals?				
Do rainy days or moldy environments make you feel unwell?				
Do you have signs of allergies (refer to the questionnaire on page 36)?				
Do you have mood swings (feeling cranky, irritable, aggressive, depressed, angry)?				
Are you hyperactive?				

Score: If you answered yes to any of the physical symptoms (questions 1 and 2) or if you answered yes or sometimes to four of the remaining questions, then you could have a fungal overgrowth requiring medical treatment.

Q. What exactly is *Candida albicans*?

A. *Candida albicans* is usually present in the digestive tract. It is a harmless yeast — harmless as long as the immune system keeps it under control. If it proliferates, candida can cause a visible skin infection and it can affect your gastrointestinal tract. Infestation is commonly referred to as candidiasis, yeast infection, or thrush. *Candida albicans* overgrowth triggers the production of IgE antibodies. (Remember: IgE is implicated in allergic reactions.) According to research published in *Clinical and Experimental Allergy*, people with atopic eczema and candidiasis are exposed to continuous IgE antibodies, which makes their eczema symptoms worse. Unbalanced gut microflora and the proliferation of fungus often come before the development of eczema. It is important to treat candida infestation immediately. The Eczema Diet is designed to minimize the risk of further infestations.

Did You Know?

Antifungal Foods
Some foods kill fungus in the gastrointestinal tract, chiefly foods from the garlic and the onion family, including eczema-safe leeks and green onions.

Worms

If you or your child is experiencing signs of worm infestation, speak to your doctor or a pharmacist about oral worming treatments — they are simple, painless, and pleasant tasting. Always wash your hands before eating to reduce the risk of worms.

Q. How do I know if I have worms?

A. We all carry some parasites in our gastrointestinal tract that can affect our health if they proliferate abnormally. Hookworms, pinworms, and whipworms can enter the intestine through the mouth or through the skin when you eat raw or unwashed food and come in contact with parasites in polluted water and soil. Signs of worm infestation include:

- grinding your teeth at night
- itchy anus, nose, or ears
- regularly wetting the bed (a child's symptom)
- frequent nosebleeds
- disturbed sleep (and/or itchy bottom at night)

If you recognize any of these signs, see your health-care provider. Most parasite infestations can be controlled with medications.

Did You Know?

What Came First?

The eczema condition or the fat abnormality? A large, carefully designed study demonstrated that the elevated omega-6 levels and other EFA abnormalities appear before the eczema manifests. This suggests that abnormal ratios of essential fatty acids in the diet and/or enzyme blockages caused by diet or stress could be involved in the onset of eczema.

Balance Your Fat Ratios

The fats you consume can affect your eczema. There are two main kinds of fat in your diet: saturated fats and unsaturated fats, which are composed of essential fatty acids (EFAs). EFAs are polyunsaturated fats that include linoleic acid (commonly known as omega-6 EFAs) and alpha-linolenic acid (known as omega-3 EFAs). In general, Western diets are far too low in omega-3 and very high in omega-6 EFAs — thanks to high intakes of margarine and vegetable oils. It has been estimated that the present Western diet ratio of omega-6 to omega-3 is 15:1 to 16:1 (instead of 1:1). This skewed ratio increases the risk of inflammation.

Guidelines for Improving Your Intestinal Health

- Speak to a pharmacist or doctor about taking a powdered oral antifungal or a topical antifungal (one that is suitable for eczema).
- If you are sexually active, your partner should also take an oral antifungal. (If he has signs of tinea cruris, otherwise known as jock itch, or if she has signs of thrush, apply a topical antifungal for 14 days and avoid sexual intercourse during this time.)
- If you have repeatedly suffered from thrush, speak to your doctor about stronger antifungal treatments.
- If you have regular bouts of candidiasis, avoid sweet foods because fungus proliferates when sugar is in the diet. Also avoid other common triggers, such as alcohol and tea.
- Take a suitable probiotic supplement (see "Probiotics," page 119).
- Ensure you are consuming lots of dietary fiber from pears, rolled oats, rice, flax seeds, buckwheat, and root vegetables, and eat 2 to 3 servings of eczema-safe grains daily (see "Eczema-Healthy Grains," page 75).
- Drink 5 to 8 glasses (48 to 64 ounces, or 1.5 to 2 L).
- Add garlic, green onions, leeks, and papaya to your diet.
- Take digestive enzymes if required.
- Chew your food properly.
- Avoid sugar and dairy products.
- Avoid drinking alcohol while you have eczema; if you have a rare special occasion when you would like to have a drink, choose eczema-safe varieties (see "Party Foods," page 153) and limit intake to 2 servings every 2 weeks.
- Avoid wheat products and other gluten-containing foods for 3 months.
- Take the amino acid glutamine if you have signs of intestinal permeability. Glutamine can help heal the gut lining, along with probiotics (page 119), B-group vitamins, vitamin E (page 111), and magnesium (page 104).
- Keep in mind that supplement therapy can fail if you continue to consume gut irritants.

Q. What are trans fats?

A. Trans fats are partially or fully hydrogenated fats that act like saturated fats and block some enzyme reactions in the body. For good health, avoid trans fats (check product packaging for phrases like "trans fats," "partially hydrogenated oil," or "hydrogenated oil"). Trans fats may be found in cheap vegetable cooking oils, doughnuts, pastries, cookies, chicken nuggets, some margarines, deep-fried foods (such as fried chicken and french fries), imitation cheese products, confectionery fats, pizza dough, and many fast foods.

The Eczema Diet shows you how to eat the correct ratios of fats by limiting omega-6 oils (no margarine and a restricted use of vegetable oils) and increasing omega-3 oils in the diet. Consuming fish, flaxseed oil, and flax seeds can increase your omega-3 intake. In this diet, saturated fat intake is lowered to decrease the amount of arachidonic acid you are consuming, so the omega-3 fats you consume can be more easily taken up by your cells.

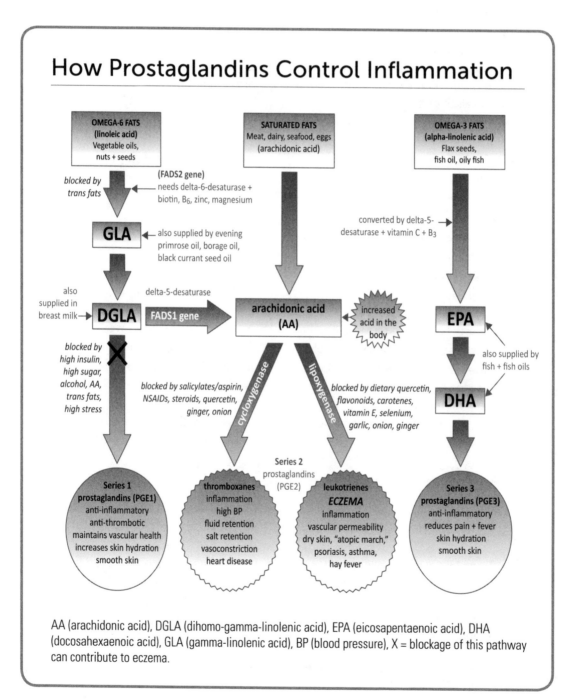

How Prostaglandins Control Inflammation

OMEGA-6 FATS (linoleic acid) Vegetable oils, nuts + seeds

SATURATED FATS Meat, dairy, seafood, eggs (arachidonic acid)

OMEGA-3 FATS (alpha-linolenic acid) Flax seeds, fish oil, oily fish

blocked by trans fats

(FADS2 gene) needs delta-6-desaturase + biotin, B6, zinc, magnesium

converted by delta-5-desaturase + vitamin C + B3

GLA ← also supplied by evening primrose oil, borage oil, black currant seed oil

also supplied in breast milk → **DGLA**

delta-5-desaturase FADS1 gene → **arachidonic acid (AA)**

increased acid in the body

EPA

also supplied by fish + fish oils

blocked by high insulin, high sugar, alcohol, AA, trans fats, high stress

X

blocked by salicylates/aspirin, NSAIDs, steroids, quercetin, ginger, onion — cycloxygenase

lipoxygenase — *blocked by dietary quercetin, flavonoids, carotenes, vitamin E, selenium, garlic, onion, ginger*

DHA

Series 1 prostaglandins (PGE1) anti-inflammatory anti-thrombotic maintains vascular health increases skin hydration smooth skin

thromboxanes inflammation high BP fluid retention salt retention vasoconstriction heart disease

Series 2 prostaglandins (PGE2)

leukotrienes *ECZEMA* inflammation vascular permeability dry skin, "atopic march," psoriasis, asthma, hay fever

Series 3 prostaglandins (PGE3) anti-inflammatory reduces pain + fever skin hydration smooth skin

AA (arachidonic acid), DGLA (dihomo-gamma-linolenic acid), EPA (eicosapentaenoic acid), DHA (docosahexaenoic acid), GLA (gamma-linolenic acid), BP (blood pressure), X = blockage of this pathway can contribute to eczema.

Q. What are prostaglandins?

A. Like polyunsaturated fats, prostaglandins can play a role in the onset of eczema. They are hormone-like substances that your body produces to moderate your hormones, your heart, your blood vessels, and your cells. They can cause or prevent skin inflammation, as in the case of eczema. Prostaglandins are grouped into three families called Series 1, 2, and 3 prostaglandins. Which series a prostaglandin falls into depends on what type of fats you eat — saturated fats or polyunsaturated omega-3 and omega-6 fats.

Q. Should I use margarine and vegetable oil instead of butter?

A. Margarines are made from vegetable oils and have been touted as a healthy alternative to butter, but research is emerging to suggest otherwise. According to a large cross-sectional study in Germany, families who predominantly use margarine (rather than butter) are more likely to have children with eczema. The frequent consumption of vegetable oils, margarine, or frying fats during the last 4 weeks of pregnancy increases the risk of having a child with eczema. So are these products as healthy as they seem? If you have a look at the ingredient panel of most margarine tubs and refined vegetable oils, you'll see they contain chemical additives, such as potassium sorbate, and research shows many food preservatives cause a worsening of eczema symptoms in more than 50% of eczema sufferers. Margarines also usually contain artificial colors (which 40% of eczema sufferers will react to) and antioxidants (which can worsen symptoms in 21% of eczema sufferers). Furthermore, margarines and vegetable oils contain large quantities of omega-6. Despite the marketing hype about the health benefits of margarine and vegetable oils, the fact is, the typical Western diet is far too rich in omega-6. Our diets are severely lacking in omega-3 (from seafood, wild/game meats, flax seeds, and walnuts), and this disrupts essential fatty acid balance and may partly explain why margarines and vegetable oils increase the risk of eczema.

Did You Know?

Omega Research

In the 1930s, researchers initially thought that omega-6 was deficient in eczema sufferers. However, research published in the 1980s confirmed the opposite: eczema sufferers tend to have elevated omega-6 in their blood and adipose tissue, in conjunction with a decrease in omega-6 metabolites, such as DGLA (dihomo-gamma-linolenic acid). When the breastmilk of nursing mothers was tested, those with elevated levels of omega-6 and low levels of DGLA in their milk had children who later went on to develop eczema.

Guidelines for Balancing Your Fat Ratios

- To promote proper functioning of the enzyme that converts omega-6 (via the FADS2 gene), consume the nutrients biotin, vitamin B6, magnesium, and zinc.
- To promote the conversion of DGLA into skin-smoothing prostaglandins, reduce stress if necessary, avoid consuming trans fats and alcohol, and limit the consumption of high-glycemic-index (GI) foods, such as white bread.
- Take the mineral chromium to reduce high insulin levels after the consumption of carbohydrates.
- Avoid margarine and foods containing margarine, such as pastries and baked goods.
- Limit the amount and types of vegetable oils in your diet (refer to "Guidelines for Selecting Cooking Oils" on page 73).
- To increase omega-3 EFA intake, eat eczema-safe fish once or twice a week (see "Safe Seafood," page 69) and eat flax seeds or use flaxseed oil five times a week (see "Flax Seeds," page 67). If you are eating fish and flax seeds, it is optional to take a fish oil supplement (eicosapentaenoic acid, or EPA, and docosahexaenoic acid, or DHA) (see "Essential Fatty Acids," page 117).
- Reduce saturated fat intake. You can enjoy lean cuts of lamb, veal, turkey, and chicken (cut the fat off meats and eat red meat no more than twice a week).
- Avoid foods containing trans fats, as well as sausages, deli meats, beef, pork, and roast crackling.
- Reduce stress, worry, and anxiety, or seek counseling for ways to cope with stress, grief, or trauma.
- Greatly reduce omega-6 EFAs in the diet.
- Don't bother taking an evening primrose oil supplement unless you find it significantly helps your skin (instead, focus on promoting DGLA conversion).
- Take a supplement containing biotin, vitamin B6, zinc, and magnesium for delta-6-desaturase enzyme reactions (so the FADS2 gene is more likely to work).
- Take a supplement containing vitamin C and vitamin B3 for delta-5-desaturase enzyme reactions (so the FADS1 gene is more likely to work), as well as quercetin and vitamin E.
- Eat garlic, leeks, and green onions.
- Favor low-GI foods to reduce insulin production and promote DGLA conversion.

Promote Liver Detoxification

The Eczema Diet recipes supply the nutrients required for liver detoxification, namely the antioxidants vitamin C, vitamin E, quercetin, and alpha-lipoic acid, which increase protection against the free radicals created during liver detoxification. Promoting proper liver detoxification can reverse or reduce multiple chemical sensitivities (this can take time to achieve). Although foods can supply many of the nutrients required for liver detoxification, additional supplementation is beneficial.

Liver Function

The liver is the second-largest organ in the body (after the skin) and it performs a range of important body functions that can greatly affect the appearance of your skin. Your liver filters more than 50 ounces (1.5 L) of blood per minute and receives a dual blood supply: one containing freshly oxygenated blood from the heart, and the other supplying blood from the stomach and intestines, rich with newly absorbed nutrients from your diet, as well as toxins, microbes, drugs, and hormones. The liver plays a vital role in detoxifying these substances so that the blood remains healthy, and it assists with supplying the body with nutrients for beautiful skin.

Detoxification Phases

When a medical drug is prescribed to a patient, what happens to that drug once it enters the body? Over the centuries, the study of detoxification has been undertaken by scientists to help answer this question. In the 1700s, scientists first hypothesized that after a toxin was consumed, it was transformed into a water-soluble substance and removed from the body via the urine. In 1842, this theory, using an amino acid supplement called glycine, was confirmed. In 1947, in his book *Detoxification Mechanisms*, R.T. Williams defined for the first time the two separate phases of detoxification. Today the scientific research on liver detoxification is an essential part of drug safety testing, done by pharmaceutical companies to reduce the risk of people overdosing while taking prescription drugs. This research on liver detoxification can also help you to be eczema-free.

Did You Know?

Fatty Liver Disease

Fatty liver disease (where your liver accumulates fat and enlarges) occurs commonly among eczema patients. According to research at the Department of Pediatrics and Allergy at Ujitakeda Hospital in Kyoto (Japan), more than 17% of non-obese children with eczema also have fatty liver. This result is significant when compared to 3.2% of non-atopic children, 3.7% of hay fever sufferers, and 5% of asthma sufferers who have fatty liver. This research showed that atopic eczema is also associated with fat malabsorption, nutritional deficiencies, and eating trans fats, all of which can affect liver health.

Phase 1 Liver Detoxification

Most drugs and food chemicals are processed through a Phase 1 reaction involving cytochrome P450 enzymes. Their role is to make toxic substances water-soluble so they can be further processed during Phase 2 of liver detoxification. Williams found that in some cases during Phase 1 liver detoxification, chemicals could become more toxic than the original substances (he thought the term detoxification could be misleading in these instances). The findings were of great importance because, before this time, therapeutic agents (such as pharmaceutical drugs) were being prescribed without doctors being aware of the metabolic fate of the drug once a patient had swallowed it. Malfunctioning Phase 1 or Phase 2 liver detoxification reactions have been implicated in adverse reactions to drugs. Food and chemical sensitivities can indicate that your Phase 1 and/or Phase 2 detoxification pathways are imbalanced.

Phase 1 can greatly increase free radical production, which can damage DNA and cause genetic mutations if your diet is not rich in antioxidants. When Phase 1 detoxification is high, you can experience an exacerbation of symptoms and you may feel lethargic. It is around this time that antihistamine drugs are often prescribed.

Did You Know?

·······················

Natural Antihistamines

Vitamin C, vitamin B6, and quercetin are natural antihistamines that have been shown in studies to prevent histamine toxicity.

Antihistamine Medications

Antihistamine medications can make you temporarily feel better because they can mask the symptoms, but there is a catch: antihistamine medications temporarily block Phase 1 liver detoxification. Blocking liver detoxification reactions creates an increased workload for your kidneys and your skin because both are left with the task of chemical waste elimination.

Although antihistamine drugs can be useful in emergencies, there are natural alternatives to antihistamine drugs that can be used on a daily basis. You can also help to minimize the potentially damaging effects of Phase 1 by consuming the dietary antioxidants vitamin C, vitamin E, quercetin, and alpha-lipoic acid.

Phase 1 Blockers

Phase 1 detoxification is reduced by antihistamine drugs, benzodiazepines (anti-anxiety drugs), ketoconazole (an antifungal drug), fluconazole (an antifungal drug, brand name Diflucan), erythromycin (an antibiotic), acid blockers (anti-ulcer medications), grapefruit (it contains a compound called naringenin, which reduces cytochrome P450 activity), and the liver-protective herb milk thistle. Although short-term blockage of Phase 1 can be useful to temporarily relieve symptoms, long-term use of these substances can be problematic because reduced liver detoxification function can burden the kidneys.

Phase 2 Detoxification

Instead of blocking Phase 1 detoxification, there is a much healthier solution: boost Phase 2 detoxification. In Phase 2, a toxin that has been partly processed in Phase 1 joins with a substance, such as an amino acid, so it can be safely removed via the urine or bile. For example, eczema sufferers are often sensitive to salicylates, which can worsen eczema symptoms.

Salicylate Removal

During Phase 2 detoxification, between 55% and 60% of dietary salicylates are joined with the amino acid glycine, allowing salicylates to be removed from the body. This is one of the reasons why glycine is effective at reducing eczema symptoms. Without this glycine-joining step, salicylates can re-enter the bloodstream and accumulate, leading to salicylate sensitivity. Preservatives, toxic heavy metals, histamines, amines, and other chemicals, both natural and artificial, are also processed during Phase 2 liver detoxification.

Q. What is chelation therapy?

A. "Chelation" means "to grab" or "to bind." Chelation therapy is a chemical process designed to remove from the body toxic heavy metals and minerals, such as lead, copper, aluminum, iron, and mercury. A binding solution is injected into the blood circulatory system that grabs heavy metals and carries them in the urine to be excreted. Reports on the effectiveness of chelation therapy are mixed, and safety is a concern. Do not try to treat yourself. Work with physicians who are well trained in using this therapy.

Liver Detoxification Questionnaire

The following questionnaire highlights other symptoms that can indicate your liver detoxification function needs dietary support. This questionnaire is suitable for adults and children. If you have a baby with eczema, you can use this questionnaire to assess maternal diet (the diet of the mother during pregnancy and breastfeeding and/or the diet of both parents before conception). Use a checkmark to highlight the answer that best suits your experience (yes = weekly or daily; sometimes = monthly or occasionally; no = never or rarely; unsure = not known).

SYMPTOMS	Yes	Sometimes	No	Unsure
Do you have any of the following?				
Dry and/or itchy skin				
Intolerance (e.g., diarrhea or feeling unwell) to greasy foods or after taking omega-3 supplements				
Foul-smelling stools				
Headaches after eating				
Hypoglycemia, low blood sugar, fatigue/energy crashes, or sleepiness after eating				
Cravings for stimulants (e.g., coffee, chocolate, sweets)				
Constipation				
Pale/grayish/dull-looking skin				
Bad breath or unpleasant body odor				
Yellow in whites of eyes				
Pain in right side under rib cage				
Water retention, or edema				
Sour taste in mouth				
High blood cholesterol: cholesterol over 200 mg/dL (American) or 5.5 mmol/L (Canadian)				
A history of jaundice				
Hepatitis				
Nausea				
Depression, moodiness, fluctuating moods				
Allergies, hives, hay fever, high blood histamine level, or dark rings under the eyes (allergic shiners)				
Gallstones				
Chronic fatigue syndrome, fibromyalgia				
Intolerance to alcohol, antibiotics, or drugs				

SYMPTOMS	Yes	Sometimes	No	Unsure
Intolerance to aspirin, salicylates, or baby teething gel				
Chemical/food sensitivities				
Sulfite sensitivity (sensitivity to wine, dried fruit, and vinegar)				

Score: If you have fewer than two of these symptoms, then taking supplements would be optional (but highly recommended) while on the Eczema Diet. If you answered yes to three or more questions, you should take supplements while on the Eczema Diet. If you have eczema, it is a sign that Phase 1 and Phase 2 are imbalanced and nutritional support is required.

Guidelines for Promoting Liver Detoxification

- To help reverse or prevent fatty liver: limit or avoid drinking alcohol, maintain a healthy weight, reduce fat intake, and add lecithin to your diet. Lecithin contains choline, which breaks down fats so they don't accumulate in the liver (see "Soy Lecithin Granules," page 71).
- Avoid trans fats.
- Prevent or reverse nutritional deficiencies with supplementation.
- Take liver detoxification nutrients to promote healthy liver function.
- Consume the nutrients required for Phase 2 liver detoxification function.
- Consume the antioxidants vitamin C, vitamin E, quercetin, and alpha-lipoic acid.
- Reduce intake of salicylates, amines, and histamine-rich foods because they create a heavy workload for your liver, kidneys, and skin.

Nutrients for Phase 2 Liver Detoxification

Your liver is the body's main chemical-processing organ to remove chemicals, histamines, and toxins. No drug can ever replace the nutrients required for liver detoxification of these substances. A healthy diet and antioxidants support liver function. What are the specific nutrients needed for liver detoxification of chemicals? Here is the list.

Sensitivities/Adverse Reactions	Phase 2 Detoxification Pathway	Nutrients and Foods Required
Amines (e.g., from meat, frozen fish, deli meats, nitrosamines) Fungal toxins Pickled foods High estrogen	Glucuronidation (metabolizes 33% of drugs, such as acetaminophen and NSAIDs, and deactivates sex hormones, especially estrogens, and food estrogens)	Magnesium, zinc, B-group vitamins, ground turmeric (spice), essential fatty acids (omega-3) (Plus, reduce dietary amines)
Histamines Histamine toxicity	Other mechanisms	Vitamin C, vitamin B_6, quercetin, taurine, methionine, cysteine, possibly magnesium and coenzyme Q10 (may need to reduce calcium intake)
Pesticide exposure Toxic heavy metals Penicillin Alcohol Acetaminophen	Glutathionylation (anti-aging if it works well)	Brussels sprouts, cabbage (and other cruciferous vegetables), glycine, glutamine, cysteine, methionine, vitamin B_2, vitamin B_6, vitamin C, selenium, glutathione (Plus, avoid toxic heavy metals)
Salicylates (salicylic acids, aspirin, teething gel) MSG (e.g., tomatoes, flavor-enhanced savory foods, such as chips) Sulfites (additives in dried fruit, wine, vinegar) Tartrazine (yellow food coloring) Preservatives	Glycination	Glycine, magnesium, taurine, vitamin B_6 and reduced salicylates
Food histamines Sulfites	Sulfation	Molybdenum (cofactor for sulfur oxidase), vitamin B_{12}, vitamin B_6, folic acid/folate, sulfur-containing foods (e.g., garlic, onion, and cabbage) Avoid additives, preserved meats, deli meats, pickled foods, vinegar, dried fruits, alcohol (especially wine)

Restore Your Acid-Alkaline Balance

There is another way to help your liver detoxify problematic chemicals: by consuming foods that have an alkalizing effect in the body. Do you remember learning about acids and bases at school? Your food does more than stop the hunger pangs and boost your energy; once your meal is digested, it releases either an acidic or an alkaline base into your bloodstream. The Eczema Diet shows how to create acid-alkaline-balanced meals that are nutritious and beneficial for your eczema. Keeping your diet in acid-alkaline balance promotes healthy blood and strong bones — and it gives your skin a healthy glow.

Acidifying Diets

The standard Western diet is unbalanced because it largely consists of acid-producing ingredients. Modern diets are generally high in protein and refined grains and low in alkalizing vegetables. It is well documented that these diets cause chronic, low-grade metabolic acidosis that worsens with age as kidney function declines.

What happens when your daily diet is constantly acid-producing? Let's say you consume a hamburger containing beef, bacon, ketchup, and lettuce, and you wash it down with a glass of diet cola or a cup of coffee. Once digested, this meal floods acids into your bloodstream and your body responds by releasing calcium (which is alkaline) into your bloodstream. This usually ensures the blood's pH returns to alkaline. This is an important process that keeps you alive.

Is the problem solved? Not exactly. Your meal has depleted some of your calcium stores, and where does your body get calcium from? Calcium can be taken from the body's reserves and leached from your bones. Excess acids can be excreted via the skin, lungs, and kidneys, which can burden these systems. Acids can be stored in your tissues, which can make the skin itchy. Research shows the consumption of Western acidifying diets causes weakened bones, muscle wasting, kidney stone formation, and damage to the kidneys.

> **Did You Know?**
>
> **Potential of Hydrogen**
>
> The measurement called pH means "potential of hydrogen," and on the pH scale, 0 is strongly acidic, 7 is neutral, and up to 14 is strongly alkaline. Your blood needs to be slightly alkaline at a pH between 7.35 and 7.45 to be healthy. Your body will do all it can to keep the blood within these limits.

Salicylate sensitivity is the most common chemical sensitivity that eczema sufferers have, and in the 1950s, alkalization was used as an effective treatment for eliminating salicylates from the body. As reported in 1955 in the *Journal of Clinical Investigation*, medical staff at hospitals used alkalization to treat salicylate poisoning from accidental aspirin overdose. Alkalization also supports detoxification of chemicals, such as preservatives, amines, food colorings, and MSG. When the urine pH exceeds an alkaline reading of 7.5, more salicylates are eliminated than reabsorbed, and three times the amount of salicylates are excreted via the urine.

Alkalization

Alkalization is the term used for the administration of highly alkalizing foods or supplements for a short period of time, such as during a detoxification program. In the 1600s, the first medical experiments regarding the body's balance of acids and alkalies were conducted. Doctors used alkalization to treat a range of health problems, including gout. In the mid-1900s, the body's acid-alkaline balance became popular for its role in the detoxification of chemicals.

3-Day Cleanse

The Eczema Diet includes a gentle 3-day alkalizing cleanse, which is a liver detoxification and gastrointestinal cleansing program designed specifically for adults with eczema and chemical sensitivities. Although this is a nutritious alkalization program for short-term use, for everyday health, your daily diet needs to have acid-alkaline balance. Some of the recipes in the Eczema Diet are highly alkalizing, such as Tarzan Juice (page 207), Healthy Skin Juice (page 206), and Alkaline Bomb Salad (page 218), but most of the recipes are classified as acid-alkaline-balanced because they contain both alkalizing and healthy acid-producing ingredients so they meet your body's nutritional needs for protein, fiber, minerals, and essential fatty acids.

How to Monitor Your pH

Your pH changes throughout the day because each meal and drink influences your blood, urine, saliva, and tissue pH readings. You can test your urine and saliva pH at home, several times a day if you wish, using a pH test kit containing litmus paper (these test kits are available from some health food shops and online).

The saliva test measures your body tissue pH, and it should be done about 30 minutes after eating or drinking. When you test your urine pH (this is the preferred test), the amount of acids your kidneys are excreting is measured. It is useful to monitor your pH several times a day, for at least 2 weeks, so you can see for yourself how your diet affects your pH (also keep in mind that stress can cause an acid reading). If you note that you are particularly acidic, you can eat or drink one of the recipes included in Part 7 to help restore acid-alkaline balance.

Acid-Alkaline Balance Questionnaire

This questionnaire is suitable for adults and children. If you have a baby with eczema, you can use this questionnaire to assess maternal diet (the diet of the mother during pregnancy and breastfeeding, or the diet of both parents before conception). Monitor any foods and beverages you consume on a regular basis (or any symptom). Use a checkmark to highlight the answer that best suits your experience (yes = weekly or daily; sometimes = monthly or occasionally; no = never or rarely; unsure = not known).

SYMPTOM/BEHAVIOR	Yes	Sometimes	No	Unsure
Do you do any of the following?				
Eat fewer than 5 servings (2½ cups/625 mL) of vegetables daily?				
Eat processed deli meats and/or smoked meats?				
Drink caffeine (coffee, tea, chocolate milk) daily?				
Eat beef, sausages, and/or pork?				
Eat processed breakfast cereal?				
Add sugar to foods or drinks (e.g., coffee, tea, or cereal)?				
Eat pickled vegetables (e.g., gherkins)?				
Eat dried soup mixes?				
Eat cheese and/or sweetened fruit-flavored yogurt?				
Eat commercial ketchup or barbecue sauce?				
Eat ice cream and/or custard?				
Regularly eat corn or corn products?				
Eat lots of fruit?				
Take medical drugs or recreational drugs?				
Eat chocolate?				
Eat peanuts or peanut butter?				
Drink alcohol and/or sodas?				
Consume artificial sweetener?				
Eat white flour products (e.g., white bread, baked goods)?				
Eat desserts made from processed foods?				
Consume margarine or softened butter containing additives?				
Have regular bouts of *Candida albicans* overgrowth or yeast infection?				

Score: If you answered yes to three or more questions, your diet is likely to be acidifying and contributing to your eczema. However, if you drink a cup of coffee or tea, or a glass of alcohol or soda every day, your pH reading is likely to be highly acidic.

Guidelines for Restoring Alkaline-Acid Balance

- Aim to eat a healthy, balanced diet that contains both alkaline and nutritious acid-forming foods.
- Keep in mind that it is not necessary, or recommended, to follow a 100% alkalizing diet for more than a week at a time. There are many acid-forming foods, such as legumes and whole grains, which are important for healthy skin, and if you like eating meat, you can enjoy it in moderation (with the fat carefully cut off or drained).
- If you can avoid red meat and favor legumes, skinless chicken, and eczema-safe varieties of fish, this would be ideal.
- Drink a glass of Tarzan Juice (page 207) or Healthy Skin Juice (page 206), or eat Alkaline Bomb Salad (page 218) daily, because they are strongly alkalizing.
- Avoid alcoholic drinks because they are highly acid-forming.

Quick Reference Acid-Alkaline Food Guide

Alkalizing Food	Acidifying Food
- Vegetables - Herbs - Sprouts - Rice malt syrup - Apple cider vinegar - Few fruits (banana, lemon, lime) - Water, pure spring - Neutral: filtered water	- Meat, seafood, beans, legumes (protein) - Grains - Corn - Peanuts - Most fruits - Sugar - Sweeteners - Artificial additives - Sodas - Alcohol - Caffeine products - Vinegars (except apple cider vinegar)

Stage 1 Alkalizing and Acidifying Foods

When selecting food items that will help you restore acid-alkaline balance, refer to the Eczema-Safe Food Guidelines (pages 174–182). These provide information not only on the acidity and alkalinity of foods but also on their salicylate, sulfite, amine, glycemic-index, gluten, and additive content.

Bad Lunch/Good Lunch

Acidifying foods often appear to be healthy, but if they are not balanced with alkalizing foods, they can intensify eczema symptoms.

Here are some examples of lunch box meals that are acidifying and overloaded with chemicals that can aggravate eczema symptoms:

Lunch box 1: This meal includes a whole-grain sandwich using bread to suit your allergies, strawberries, an additive-free muesli (granola) bar, and organic fruit yogurt.

✗ Why is this lunch box a bad choice? This lunch box seems healthy, but every item is acid-producing and nothing is alkalizing. This lunch could cause a flare-up of eczema symptoms thanks to the natural chemicals present in the fruits.

Lunch box 2: This meal includes a ham sandwich on white bread with margarine, an orange, cheese, fruit-flavored yogurt, cake or cookies, and chocolate milk.

✗ Why is this lunch box a bad choice? Every item is strongly acid-producing and overloaded with irritating chemicals. This lunch box would cause your eczema to flare up (and it could be severe).

Here are some examples of eczema-safe lunch boxes:

Lunch box 3: This meal includes a whole-grain salad sandwich using bread to suit your allergies, iceberg lettuce, grated carrot, and mung bean sprouts; a pear muffin (homemade); plain rice crackers; baked banana chips (homemade); celery sticks; and filtered water.

✓ Why is this lunch box a good choice? Celery and salad ingredients are alkalizing and sprouts are strongly alkalizing (bonus points for this item), the other foods are healthy acid-producing items, and filtered water is neutral.

Lunch box 4: This meal includes an organic chicken and lettuce wrap (using spelt bread or flatbread), a banana, carrot sticks, brown rice crackers, and filtered water.

✓ Why is this lunch box a good choice? Carrot, lettuce, and banana are alkalizing. The chicken, bread, and crackers are acid-forming, but they are also eczema-safe and supply nutrients for a balanced diet.

Stage 1 Alkalizing
and Acidifying Foods

Part 2

Eczema-Healthy Foods

Chapter 3
Top 20 Eczema-Healthy Foods

The Eczema Diet is relatively easy to start and to keep going without relapse into eczema-aggravating habits. If you avoid specific foods that aggravate eczema and replace them with eczema-healthy foods, you should be able to control your symptoms or your child's — and even reverse them.

The top 20 eczema-healthy foods supply valuable nutrients to help decrease inflammation and promote skin repair and maintenance. This list of safe foods includes references to the recipes in this book, as well as some handy food preparation tips.

1. Banana

Although most other fruits are acid-forming and rich in problematic chemicals, regular bananas have unique alkalizing properties, thanks to their high potassium content. Bananas are salicylate-free, with the exception of sugar bananas (lady fingers), which should be avoided. They are a fiber-rich and nutritious energy snack. Although they contain some amines, they also supply their own amine- and histamine-lowering nutrients, magnesium and vitamin C, so this nutrient-dense snack should not pose a problem for those who are mildly sensitive to amines.

Preparation: Have a banana as a snack, prepare one in the Healthy Skin Smoothie (page 209), freeze them to make ice pops, or treat yourself to sliced banana on Spelt Pancakes (page 201).

Rules of Thumb for the Eczema Diet Servings

1. Eat 5 servings of eczema-healthy vegetables daily.
2. Eat 2 servings of eczema-healthy fruit daily.
3. Eat at least 2 servings of eczema-healthy grains daily.
4. Eat 2 servings of eczema-healthy protein daily.
5. Drink 5 to 8 glasses, or 48 to 64 ounces (1.5 to 2 L), of filtered water daily (including eczema-healthy vegetable juices and soups).

(A serving equals $\frac{1}{2}$ cup/125 mL, so 5 servings of vegetables is approximately $2\frac{1}{2}$ cups/625 mL.)

Refer to the Eczema-Safe Food Guidelines (pages 174–182) for examples of these eczema-safe foods.

2. Papaya

Papaya is a red fruit that provides a range of carotenoids, which are potent antioxidants for modulating gene activity to protect against inflammatory damage and tumor growth. The lycopene content in papaya helps to protect the skin from sun damage and is a rich source of vitamin C, the antihistamine vitamin, which can help allergy sufferers manage their symptoms. Papaya contains the digestive enzyme papain, which is used in some digestive supplements to aid protein digestion. Papain may kill parasites in the gut. After antibiotic use or a bout of illness, you can eat a serving of papaya daily to promote recolonization of beneficial bacteria in the gastrointestinal tract.

Preparation: Papaya is usually eaten raw, with the skin and seeds removed. The seeds contain potent antimicrobial properties and they can be eaten to flush worms out of the bowel ("flush" being the operative word because they can cause severe diarrhea, so use with caution and do not give children papaya seeds). Eating papaya flesh does not cause diarrhea, although the fruit does contain a moderate amount of amines, so if you are highly sensitive to amines, make sure you are also taking a vitamin C, B6, and quercetin supplement.

Recipes: Papaya Rice Paper Rolls (page 222), Spelt Pancakes (page 201), Healthy Skin Smoothie (page 209), and Surprise Porridge (page 199).

> After antibiotic use or a bout of illness, you can eat a serving of papaya daily to promote recolonization of beneficial bacteria in the gastrointestinal tract.

3. Beef or Chicken Broth

A well-made broth soothes the gastrointestinal tract and provides the skin-repairing amino acid glycine. Glycine is needed to produce connective tissue and enhances detoxification of chemicals. Broth contains collagen, calcium, and magnesium, and for those in poor health or suffering from a cold or flu, sipping cysteine-rich broth throughout the day can reduce mucus and offer relief. Its content of chondroitin sulfate and hyaluronan helps to lubricate joints, making broth valuable for arthritis sufferers. A regular store-bought broth will not do, however. For a steaming cup of broth to be both a food and a "medicine," it must be made correctly — there is a trick to extracting the nutrients from the bones and this step cannot be skipped.

Preparation: Broth is made by adding vegetables and bones (that have a little bit of meat, cartilage, and tendons left on them) to a pot with plenty of water. The addition of a weak acid causes an acid-base chemical reaction and the alkaline minerals are drawn right out of the bones (similar to when you eat an acid-forming Western diet that slowly leaches calcium from your bones). Eczema-safe acids include ascorbic acid (pure vitamin C powder) and citric acid (from the baking section of larger supermarkets or pharmacies).

Although the cooking time is extensive (a minimum of 6 hours for a nutrient-dense broth), the good news is that broth is an inexpensive meal. You can use a chicken carcass or beef bones and other bones that the local butcher usually discards or sells cheaply (not pork bones, though). Beef bones that have been roasted in the oven make for a deliciously aromatic broth.

Recipes: Therapeutic Broth (page 212). Vegetarians and vegans can alternatively make Alkaline Veggie Broth (page 214).

4. Potato

> An eczema sufferer needs to avoid many foods, so it is comforting to know you can enjoy a side of mashed potato and homemade potato wedges.

An eczema sufferer needs to avoid many foods, so it is comforting to know you can enjoy a side of mashed potato and homemade potato wedges. The humble potato is a valuable staple food, rich in fiber, potassium, and vitamin C. One medium white potato contains a whopping 600 mg of potassium, making it one of the few carbohydrate-rich foods that are alkalizing. A medium potato also contains vitamin B_6 for the detoxification of chemicals, such as salicylates, alpha-lipoic acid for potent antioxidant protection, and 30 mg of vitamin C, which is enough to stave off scurvy.

Most white potatoes have a high to medium glycemic index. Sweet potato has a lower glycemic index than most varieties of white potatoes, making it suitable for people with diabetes and those with energy problems. It is anti-inflammatory and contains some salicylates. A cup (250 mL) of mashed sweet potato contains 950 mg of alkalizing potassium, 11,520 mcg of antioxidant beta-carotene, 76 mg of calcium, 54 mg of magnesium, 33 mg of histamine-lowering vitamin C, and 26 mg of choline to guard against fatty liver conditions.

Recipes: Smashed Potatoes (page 232), Chickpea Casserole (page 224), Roasted Sweet Potato Salad (page 219), Baked Fish with Mash (page 225), Teething Rusks (page 204), Easy Roast Chicken (page 228), Sunshine Soup (page 216), and New Potato and Leek Soup (page 215).

5. Buckwheat

Buckwheat is used as a gluten-free grain, though it is actually an herb seed. Buckwheat is available roasted and as groats, flour, pasta, and tea. The flour can be made into pancakes or added to gluten-free muffin mixes. Unlike wheat, it is gentle on the digestive tract and rich in the potent antioxidant flavonoids rutin and quercetin. In experiments, rutin has been found to prevent capillary fragility and high blood pressure. Quercetin lowers the blood histamine level and it has a strong anti-inflammatory effect because it inhibits leukotrienes, which are produced during an eczema flare-up. Although buckwheat flour is not as potent as quercetin, it supplies dietary fiber and is a nutritious way to add skin-repairing nutrients into your diet.

Although buckwheat flour is not as potent as quercetin, it supplies dietary fiber and is a nutritious way to add skin-repairing nutrients into your diet.

Recipes: Buckwheat Crêpes (page 202) and Chicken with Green Beans (page 230).

6. Mung Bean Sprouts

Mung bean sprouts are like little alkalizing "bombs" when added to your meals. They are one of the few strongly alkalizing foods available. They contain magnesium, vitamin K, folate, potassium, and vitamin C, and they are salicylate-free. Mung bean sprouts must be eaten fresh and used up quickly (check use-by dates and don't buy sprouts that don't have a visible use-by date or a "packed" date listed). Wash them thoroughly in a bowl of water before use.

Preparation: Sprouting your own mung beans is easy (see page 66). Add them to salads and savory dishes, and they make a healthy addition to children's snacks (kids might prefer them served without the green shells).

Recipes: Design Your Own Sandwich (page 223), Roasted Sweet Potato Salad (page 219), Roasted Potato Snack (page 244), Papaya Rice Paper Rolls (page 222), and Tarzan Juice (page 207).

Sprouting Recipe

Serves: 4

- Preparation time: 5 minutes
- Soaking time: overnight
- Rinse and drain twice daily for 2 days

You can use this recipe to sprout mung beans, spelt grains, barley, or lentils, which are your eczema-safe choices for sprouting. If you use lentils, they must not be "split" lentils or they won't sprout. Whole spelt grains are available from health food shops — they may be hard to find — and they can be used to make sprouted spelt bread. In Stage 2, you can also sprout dried green peas. They are lovely when sprouted.

⅓ cup	dried mung beans	75 mL
1	wide glass jar or container	1
	Filtered water	
1	cheesecloth or mesh to cover	1
1	elastic band	1

- Rinse the mung beans before use and remove any damaged ones that look darker or split. After rinsing them, place them into a glass jar or container.

- Fill the jar with lukewarm water to help soften hard beans and cover the jar with a piece of breathable cheesecloth or mesh and secure with an elastic band.

- Set aside on the kitchen counter in low light, away from direct sunlight and not in a dark cupboard. Soak them overnight.

- The next morning, drain off the excess water and rinse with more water. (If using cheesecloth, remove the cloth, keep the beans in the jar, fill the jar with water, place a mesh strainer over the top, and drain the water. If using mesh, keep the beans in the jar and the mesh on top, and rinse.)

- Rinse and drain twice daily for at least 2 days. For little mung bean sprouts, rinse and drain every 8 to 12 hours for 2 to 3 days. Larger sprouts will take 4 to 5 days and you'll need to continue the rinsing routine so they don't dry out.

- As soon as the sprouts are ready, drain any excess water, dry them, and store them, wrapped in a paper towel (or something to soak up the excess moisture), in an airtight container in the refrigerator.

- Use them within 4 days for maximum freshness.

7. Oats

Eczema sufferers need to start their day with a nutritious breakfast. Whole-grain or rolled oats provide more dietary fiber and protein than other grain cereals. They are a source of vitamin E, zinc, potassium, iron, manganese, and silica, an essential mineral for strengthening connective tissue in the skin. Oats contain soluble fiber — when they are made into porridge, it appears gluey during cooking. The fiber is valuable for gastrointestinal health, helping to lower cholesterol and cleanse pathogens and toxin-loaded bile from the bowel.

Pure oats are gluten-free, but because of cross-contamination from being grown and processed alongside wheat, they may have gluten. Gluten-free oats are available but often hard to find, so alternatively you can soak your oats overnight to make the gluten easier to digest. This also reduces the phytic acid content.

Recipes: Omega Muesli (page 198), New Anzac Cookies (page 250), and Surprise Porridge (page 199). If you are gluten intolerant, make Quinoa Porridge (page 200) as an alternative.

Pure oats are gluten-free, but because of cross-contamination from being grown and processed alongside wheat, they may have gluten.

8. Flax Seeds

Flax seeds, also known as linseeds, are small brown seeds best known for their rich content of anti-inflammatory omega-3 essential fatty acids. The seeds are a source of phytochemicals, silica, mucilage, oleic acid, protein, vitamin E, and dietary fiber for gastrointestinal and liver health. Flaxseed oil contains more than 50% omega-3 essential fatty acids.

Omega-3 is highly unstable. It is easily damaged by heat, and once the seeds have been processed into oil or ground into a fine powder, they can go rancid if not stored correctly. For these reasons, do not buy pre-ground flax seeds or a ground mixture of flax, sunflower, and almond (LSA), and don't purchase flaxseed oil that has not been refrigerated in the shop. Flaxseed oil must not be heated or used for frying, and should be refrigerated at all times.

Preparation: *How to grind flax seeds*: Place whole flax seeds into a coffee or seed grinder and grind them to a fine powder. Grind flax seeds weekly to ensure freshness and store them in a sealed glass container in the refrigerator.

Recipes: Whole or finely ground flax seeds can be mixed into porridge (Omega Muesli, page 198) or sprinkled onto fruit (Eczema-Safe Fruit Salad, page 246). Flaxseed oil can be used in Healthy Skin Smoothie (page 209) and in Stage 2 with Omega Salad Dressing (page 220).

Recommended Daily Amounts of Flaxseed by Age

Drink plenty of water when eating flax seeds because the fiber absorbs about five times the weight of the seed.

Age	Daily Amount
Adult	2 to 4 teaspoons (10 to 20 mL) ground flax seeds daily or 2 to 3 teaspoons (10 to 15 mL) flaxseed oil daily
5–17 years	1 to 2 teaspoons (5 to 10 mL) ground flax seeds daily or ½ teaspoon (2 mL) flaxseed oil daily
1–4 years	½ to 1 teaspoon (2 to 5 mL) ground flax seeds daily or ¼ teaspoon (1 mL) flaxseed oil daily

9. Brussels Sprouts

Don't groan. I used to hate Brussels sprouts until I found out the amazing health benefits they possess. Brussels sprouts are alkalizing and offer a unique and powerful combination of nutrients, including loads of vitamin C as well as potassium, folate, choline, and dietary fiber. They contain a valuable antioxidant, alpha-lipoic acid, which regenerates vitamin C and vitamin E, lowers blood sugar levels, and increases the formation of anti-aging glutathione to boost liver detoxification.

Like cabbage, Brussels sprouts are a cruciferous vegetable from the mighty brassica family and are rich in anti-cancer indoles. To retain more of the health benefits, favor steaming Brussels sprouts over frying or boiling.

Recipes: Baked Fish with Mash (page 225), Therapeutic Broth (page 212), and New Potato and Leek Soup (page 215).

10. Green Onions

Green onions, also referred to as scallions and shallots, are part of the onion family, and like the onion, green onions contain histamine-lowering, anti-inflammatory quercetin. Like garlic (but in lower concentrations), green onions possess antioxidant flavonoids that convert to allicin when cut or crushed. Lab experiments show that allicin helps liver cells to reduce cholesterol and has antibacterial, antiviral, and antifungal properties. Green onions contain folate, vitamin C, beta-carotene, and lutein. They are one of the richest sources of vitamin K, which is vital for healthy skin. Just 1½ oz (50 g) of raw green onions provides 103 mcg of vitamin K, nearly double the daily adequate intake for adults.

Recipes: Chickpea Rice (page 234), Country Chicken Soup (page 217), and Sticks and Stones (page 226).

11. Fish

High fish intake during pregnancy is associated with a decreased risk of eczema. Fish is a good source of protein, vitamin D, and iodine. Studies show 2 to 3 servings of fish each week are beneficial for elevating mood and increasing the health of the brain, skin, and heart. Good sources of omega-3, EPA, and DHA include trout, salmon, sardines, herring, and fish oil supplements. Other minor sources of EPA and DHA include low-fat seafood, such as carp, pike, haddock, oysters, clams, scallops, and squid. It is important to favor eczema-safe fish, which are low in mercury.

Recipes: Sticks and Stones (page 226), Roasted Potato Snack (page 244), and Baked Fish with Mash (page 225).

Safe Seafood

These seafoods are low in mercury, as is the case with all small-sized fish (if in doubt, ask your local fishmonger at the fish shop). The general rule is: the higher up the food chain and the bigger the fish, the more mercury it may contain.

- Bream
- Catfish
- Dory (small fillets)
- Flounder
- Hake
- Herring
- Lobster
- Oysters
- Salmon (except for smoked salmon)
- Sardines
- Shrimp
- Trout and rainbow trout
- Tuna in springwater or brine

Guidelines for Safe Seafood

- You can make a healthy snack with 3 ounces (95 g) of canned tuna once a week. Canned light tuna is sourced from smaller-sized tuna.
- Salmon and trout are commonly farmed in Western countries, and it has been suggested that these fish contain fewer nutrients than fish fresh from the ocean. However, if you cannot buy ocean-caught fish, farmed fish is an acceptable source.

continued...

Fish to Avoid

Trout, sardines, canned tuna, and salmon are rich in amines. Do not consume amine-rich fish more than once a week and discontinue use if you have an adverse reaction.

These fish often contain high levels of mercury and should be avoided. If you eat a serving of mercury-rich fish, health authorities recommend you should then avoid eating all seafood for at least 2 weeks to allow time for your body to detoxify the mercury.

- Cod (large fillets)
- King mackerel
- Marlin
- Perch (orange roughy)
- Snapper (larger fillets)
- Swordfish
- Tuna (larger fillets, albacore, southern bluefin)

Guidelines

- Do not eat frozen fish because it is 10 times higher in histamines.
- Avoid prawns and shrimp because they are treated with a sulfite preservative (cooked prawns and shrimp may be preservative-free, but you will need to check).
- While you have eczema, avoid smoked salmon and other smoked fish because they are highly acidifying and may contain chemicals and increased amines.
- Both adults and children can eat low-mercury fish twice a week, the portion being no bigger than the palm of your hand.
- Do not eat seafood more than three times a week because overconsumption of seafood may eventually lead to mercury accumulation.

12. Beets

Beets are an important vegetable for eczema sufferers because they have strong alkalizing properties that boost the liver's detoxification of salicylates and other chemicals. Although they contain moderate salicylates, they are abundant in antioxidants, folate, and iron. Beets are a potent blood cleanser, and research shows that beet consumption lowers blood pressure and has an aspirin-like effect, reducing the risk of blood clots.

Preparation: Grate peeled fresh beets into salads or salad sandwiches and use beets in freshly made vegetable juices. Do not consume canned beets because they contain vinegar.

Recipes: Healthy Skin Juice (page 206) and Design Your Own Sandwich (page 223), plus you can add grated beets to Alkaline Bomb Salad (page 218).

13. Soy Lecithin Granules

Lecithin is a phospholipid made up of essential fatty acids, phosphorous, inositol, and choline, which is an important component of bile, a substance the liver makes to remove unwanted chemicals and fats from the body. Lecithin helps the body to utilize fats correctly (making it ideal for eczema sufferers with abnormal fat metabolism). It is essential for liver function and helps to lower cholesterol. A healthy body produces small amounts of lecithin and it is present in protein foods, such as meats, fish, soy, and eggs. High-fat diets increase the need for lecithin, and if you don't consume enough lecithin, fatty liver can result.

Store-bought lecithin granules, made from soy, look like tiny yellow beads and have a pleasant malty flavor. Egg lecithin is also available, but it contains predominantly saturated fat, and eczema sufferers are more likely to be allergic to eggs, so this form is not recommended.

Total Daily Intake of Choline

Age Range	Serving Size	Choline Content (approx.)
Adults	1 tsp (5 mL) or ¼ oz (7 g) with food	250 mg
14–18 years	3 tsp (15 mL) or ¼ oz (7 g) with food	187 mg
9–13 years	2 tsp (10 mL) or ⅛ oz (4 g) with food	125 mg
4–8 years	1 tsp (5 mL) or ¹⁄₁₆ oz (2 g) with food	62 mg
1–3 years	¼ tsp (2 mL) or ¹⁄₃₂ oz (1 g) with food	31 mg
0–12 months	Choline is supplied in breast milk (especially when the mother's health and diet are good)	Infant formula and processed infant food if child is on solids (read labels for choline content)

Preparation: A tablespoon (15 mL) of lecithin granules makes a great addition to smoothies with added flaxseed oil. The lecithin helps your body utilize the omega-3 essential fatty acids from the oil. Consume flaxseed oil with the addition of lecithin.

Recipes: Omega Muesli (page 198), and Healthy Skin Smoothie (page 209), plus the Stage 2 recipe Flaxseed Lemon Drink (page 208).

14. Rice Bran Oil

Rice bran oil is low in salicylates and, like olive oil, rice bran oil contains oleic acid and vitamin E. It also contains omega-6 essential fatty acids, which should only be consumed in moderation. Rice bran oil also has a high smoking point.

Did You Know?

Smoking Point

When choosing an oil for frying at high heat, it is important to consider the smoking point — the temperature at which the oil begins to break down and produce smoke. A smoking oil is a sign that damage is occurring, the nutrients are being destroyed, and the oil is fast becoming bad for your health. At this point, you should carefully pour off the oil (if possible), wipe the pan clean, and start again. To reduce the risk of burned oil, use a cooking oil that has a high smoking point. A basic rule is, the more "extra virgin" or unrefined an oil is, the more easily it will burn. There are some exceptions to this rule, and rice bran oil is one of them because it is relatively heat stable and its high smoking point makes it an excellent choice for baking and frying. Nevertheless, rice bran oil can burn on very high heat, so decrease the stovetop heat to medium once it has heated up.

Guide to Cooking-Oil Smoking Points

Refined safflower oil and rice bran oil are suitable for use during Stage 1 of the Eczema Diet.

Cooking Oil	Smoking Point
Refined safflower oil	510°F (266°C)
Rice bran oil	490°F (254°C)
Ghee (Indian clarified dairy butter)	485°F (252°C)
Olive oil (refined or light)	468°F (242°C)
Soy oil (refined)	460°F (238°C)
Coconut oil (refined)	450°F (232°C)
Canola oil (refined)	400°F (204°C)
Olive oil (extra virgin)	375°F (190°C)
Coconut oil (extra virgin)	350°F (177°C)
Butter	250–300°F (121–149°C)
Safflower (virgin)	225°F (107°C)

Guidelines for Selecting Cooking Oils

- While you have eczema, do not cook with olive oil, coconut oil, canola oil, or any other oil that is not on the "Eczema-Safe Food Guidelines" (pages 174–182).
- Rice bran oil can burn on very high heat, so decrease the stovetop heat to medium once it has heated up.
- Rice bran oil contains omega-6 fatty acids, so it should only be used sparingly.
- While you have eczema, a cooking oil–free diet would be the healthiest choice (this means using no cooking oil, not even rice bran oil). This may be difficult to achieve, so alternatively see if you can have some "oil-free" days (on these days, make salads or one of the soup recipes or steam veggies and have them with boiled or steamed chicken or steamed fish).

15. Rice Malt Syrup

Ideally, your diet should have no added sweeteners, but for those of you who wish to use sweeteners, the best choice is rice malt syrup, for two reasons: it is alkalizing, whereas all other sweeteners convert to acid in the body, and it is low in salicylates and other chemicals. Rice malt syrup is milder than honey, so more may be required in recipes. If you have chronic candida or fungal overgrowth, go sweetener-free. Sugar is very acid-producing and should be used only, for example, on rare occasions when you make birthday cake.

Eczema-Safe Sweeteners

In order of preference, here are the sweeteners eczema sufferers can use in recipes:

- Rice malt syrup (alkalizing, low in chemicals)
- Pure maple syrup (acid-producing, low in chemicals)
- Golden syrup (acid-producing, low in chemicals)

Sweeteners to Avoid

In general, eczema sufferers should avoid the following sweeteners because they may aggravate eczema symptoms:

- Honey
- Molasses
- Fructose
- Artificial sweeteners
- Refined white sugar (highly acid-producing)

Recipes: For those of you who have a child with eczema, do not suddenly take every sugary food out of their diet. You can offer them sweet eczema-safe alternatives, such as New Anzac Cookies (page 250) and Pear Muffins (page 203). A couple of the sweet recipes require golden syrup, which is not highly refined. If this ingredient is not available in your country, use pure maple syrup instead, but avoid using imitation maple syrup because it may contain additives. Barley malt is often used to sweeten soy milks, but this sweetener should be eczema-safe if you are not gluten intolerant. It you are allergic to gluten, use malt-free soy milk or organic rice milk because they are both gluten-free.

16. Non-Dairy Milks

Dairy products, especially animal milks (cow, goat, sheep), should be avoided by eczema sufferers. To meet your need for calcium, instead of eating dairy products, you can eat protein twice daily and consume 5 servings of alkalizing vegetables for bone health. An alkalizing diet is better at strengthening bones than dairy products. For those of you who would like to consume milk in your porridge, smoothies, and baked goods, here are the best options for you.

Organic Soy Milk

Like all processed food products, soy milk has its good and bad points. The best choice is any variety containing organic "whole" soybeans because these are high quality and less processed. Do not buy soy milk listing "soy protein isolate" in the ingredients. Soy isolate was once considered a waste product and may contain aluminum. Soy is rich in phytic acid, an anti-nutrient that binds minerals, such as zinc, which is an important nutrient for eczema sufferers. For this reason, soy milk is restricted in Stage 1 of the Eczema Diet. Soy milk contains weak estrogens (like the hormone estrogen), and a healthy diet rich in the liver detoxification nutrients magnesium, zinc, and B-group vitamins helps the body to properly detoxify estrogen (refer to "Nutrients for Phase 2 Liver Detoxification," page 54).

The ingredient barley malt, which is added to soy milks for added sweetness, contains gluten, so if you are gluten intolerant, look for malt-free soy milk or use organic rice milk. If you choose to drink soy milk or any milk, keep in mind they are processed products, so consume only in moderation (e.g., a splash on your porridge or to make creamy Smashed Potatoes, page 232). If available, choose organic soy milk that is fresh (in the refrigerated section of the supermarket), that contains added fiber and calcium, and that has a low glycemic index.

Rice Milk

Rice milk is a sweet, watery milk that is low-allergy and low in chemicals, so it is regarded as eczema-safe. If purchasing rice milk, favor organic rice milk that is "calcium fortified," which means it has added calcium. Rice milk often contains sunflower oil, which is usually eczema-safe. Although some health-care professionals tend to favor rice milk over soy milk, be aware that rice milk has a very high glycemic index, so it is not suitable for diabetics or those with hypoglycemia or energy problems of any kind. For this reason, only use rice milk in moderation and take a chromium supplement daily to promote blood sugar balance (for chromium information, see page 108).

Oat Milk

A serving of oat milk is rich in fiber, calcium, and vitamin A. If you are vegan, it is a valuable source of iron, providing 10% of the recommended dietary intake. Oat milk is lactose-free and it contains gluten, so don't use oat milk if you are allergic to wheat or gluten intolerant.

> **Did You Know?**
> ....
> **Almond Milk Caution**
> Almond milk is rich in salicylates and may cause flare-ups. It is not suitable for eczema sufferers.

17. Grains

Some grains can help relieve eczema symptoms, but others can exacerbate them.

> ## Eczema-Healthy Grains
>
> The following grains are eczema-safe because they are low in natural chemicals and contain no artificial additives. If possible, soak grains before consuming them.
>
> - Barley
> - Basmati rice
> - Brown rice (not instant)
> - Buckwheat
> - Oat bran
> - Quinoa (not puffed)
> - Rice bran
> - Rye
> - Spelt
> - Whole-grain or rolled oats (porridge)

Grains to Avoid

Wheat: The Eczema Diet is wheat-free. Going wheat-free for a few months gives the digestive tract time to repair. You might find that you are better able to tolerate wheat after having a break from it. The Eczema Diet is not gluten-free, but if you are gluten intolerant, it is easy to adapt this diet by avoiding all gluten-containing products, including wheat, spelt, rye, barley, and oats.

Corn, polenta (cornmeal), and most commercial breakfast cereals: These grains are rich in irritating chemicals, such as salicylates.

Amaranth, millet, tapioca, jasmine rice, instant/quick-cooking rice, and Japanese glutinous rice: These grains have a very high glycemic index, which triggers high insulin in the blood (for reasons why high insulin is bad for eczema, see "How Prostaglandins Control Inflammation," page 46).

Did You Know?
Grains and Phytic Acid

Grains, legumes, and nuts contain phytic acid, an anti-nutrient that reduces the absorption of zinc, copper, calcium, and iron. The traditional methods of making sourdough bread by fermenting, sprouting, and soaking grains reduce the phytic acid content, increase gluten tolerance, and make minerals more available for skin repair and maintenance. Although consuming grains, legumes, and nuts in moderation should not cause deficiencies, there is an increased risk when large quantities are consumed.

Soaking Grains

Soaking grains is optional during the Eczema Diet, but it is highly recommended. The key is to think ahead and always have a couple of bowls of grains soaking on your kitchen counter. If the counter is bare, you know it is time to soak some more grains.

Using a weak acid when soaking grains is an optional step, but it is highly recommended because it changes the pH of the water, speeding up the breakdown of phytic acid. This increases the nutritional content of the grains.

Weak acids suitable for eczema sufferers are ascorbic acid (pure vitamin C powder) and citric acid. Ascorbic acid is preferable and is readily available online and from compounding chemists. Do not use other types of vitamin C. Citric acid is usually found in the baking section in larger supermarkets and pharmacies. Although sensitivities are rare, you may be sensitive to citric acid, so if gastrointestinal disturbances occur, discontinue use. Ascorbic acid and citric acid add a lovely tangy flavor to dips and spreads and they can be used to make Therapeutic Broth (page 212).

Recipes: Sesame-Free Hummus (page 239) and Parsley Pesto (page 241).

Preparation

Grains are generally soaked overnight for use in the morning or soaked first thing in the morning if you are consuming the grains in the evening. The exceptions are barley and buckwheat, which need less than 2 hours soaking time. When soaking grains, you will need:

- Bowl or glass container
- Grains of choice
- Filtered water (room temperature or tepid)
- Clean tea towel or plastic wrap (to keep out potential bugs)
- Pinch of ascorbic acid or citric acid (optional)

1. Place your choice of grain into a bowl and cover with double the quantity of water.
2. Mix in a pinch of ascorbic acid or citric acid and cover with plastic wrap or a clean tea towel.
3. Leave on the counter away from direct sunlight (do not refrigerate or place in a dark cupboard).
4. Soak for the recommended length of time.
5. Drain off the water using a strainer and rinse with fresh water to remove the vitamin C, or ascorbic acid, flavor.
6. The grains are ready to use. Use soaked grains within 13 hours or strain, rinse, and refrigerate them until needed (use refrigerated grains within 3 days).

Grain Soaking and Cooking Times

Grain	Raw Quantity	Soaking Time	Cooking Time
Buckwheat, whole	½ cup (125 mL) per adult	At least 1 hour	10 minutes (refer to package)
Barley	1 cup (250 mL)	At least 2 hours	20 minutes if soaked, 45 minutes if not soaked
Oats, rolled (porridge)	½ cup (125 mL) per adult ⅓ cup (75 mL) per child ¼ cup (60 mL) per toddler	12 hours (overnight)	Omega Muesli (page 198); no cooking required
Quinoa (not puffed)	½ cup (125 mL) per adult ⅓ cup (75 mL) per child ¼ cup 60 mL) per toddler	12 hours (overnight)	At least 20 minutes
Rice, basmati and white	1½ cups (375 mL) (feeds a family of four)	12 hours (overnight)	7–10 minutes
Rice, brown	2½ cups (625 mL) (feeds a family of four)	12 hours (overnight)	20–25 minutes

Eczema-Safe Flours

Baking with spelt flour is preferable because the gluten makes the recipes work brilliantly, and the kids can't tell the difference. Buckwheat makes a very nutritious flour, but it is an acquired taste, best used in pancakes with rice malt syrup and sliced banana. If you need to use a packet of gluten-free flour, check for additives. Note that highly processed white cornflour is acceptable to consume in small amounts, but corn or yellow cornmeal are not eczema-safe. Because flours are highly processed or ground into a fine powder, making them fast to digest, they usually have a high-GI rating. If the flour is used in nutritious recipes containing protein, the GI may be reduced. The Eczema Diet favors buckwheat, rice, and spelt flours. If you are looking for baking helpers, use gluten-free baking powder or baking soda (also gluten-free).

- Buckwheat flour
- Rice flour or brown rice flour
- Spelt flour (whole-grain if available)
- Oat flour
- Quinoa flour
- Arrowroot flour

Eczema-Healthy Breads

If you can eat gluten, then spelt bread is the top choice for eczema sufferers.

Eczema-safe breads are generally easy to digest (or gentler on the digestive tract than wheat breads). If you can eat gluten, then spelt bread is the top choice for eczema sufferers. Spelt bread tastes similar to wheat, and spelt sourdough bread uses the traditional, non-yeast method of bread-making, making it naturally lower in phytic acid and low GI. It supplies energy slowly and does not trigger high blood insulin release.

When choosing gluten-free bread, refer to the eczema-safe grain and flour lists. If buying store-bought breads, avoid artificial preservative calcium propionate.

- Gluten-free bread (if necessary)
- Plain sprouted breads (may contain gluten)
- Rye bread (no wheat)
- Spelt Lavash Bread (flatbread)
- Spelt sourdough bread
- Sprouted spelt loaf

Recipes: Spelt recipes include Spelt Lavash Bread for making flatbread or baked into Spelt Chips (variation, page 243), Spelt Pancakes (page 201), and Pear Muffins (page 203).

18. Animal and Vegetarian Protein

Your skin, muscles, brain cells, hair, and nails need protein to function; without it, your muscles would begin to waste; your skin, hair, and nails would suffer; and your body would swell with fluid retention. Children stop growing without protein. However, if you eat too much protein — for example, if you follow a high-protein low-carb diet for too long — you can end up with muscle wasting, constipation, and an increased risk of bowel cancer, skin rashes, acne, and kidney problems. For optimal health of the skin and body, a balanced or moderate amount of protein is needed in the diet. As you choose the best protein for you, consider these recommendations:

- Eat protein from animal sources that are free-range or organic where possible.
- Remove chicken skin and cut fatty pieces off meats.
- Buy only the freshest cuts of meat.
- Buy only meats that are free of preservatives and low in fat.
- If buying ground meat, ask your butcher to grind it fresh.

Egg Caution

Because eczema sufferers are often highly allergic to eggs, you should consider avoiding eggs during Stage 1 of the Eczema Diet even if no allergy is suspected. Then during Stage 2, after your eczema has cleared up, if you are not allergic to eggs, you may like to add them back into your diet.

- Always check labels on packaged meat and fish to make sure there are no additives or preservatives.
- Do not consume meat or fish that has a strong or unpleasant odor.
- Do not consume fish that has been frozen, because it is high in amines.

Guidelines for Selecting Eczema-Healthy Protein

Protein Sources to Avoid

- Dairy products (histamine)
- Deli meats, such as salami, bacon, and ham (contain nitrates)
- Eggs (if an allergy or intolerance is suspected)
- Frozen fish (is rich in histamines)
- Frozen meats and leftovers (can be high in amines)
- Liver (is high in pesticides and vitamin A)
- Pork and beef (strongly acid-forming)
- Shrimp and prawns (are treated with sulfite preservative)
- Sausages (contain nitrates)
- Sliced/processed chicken and turkey (contain flavor enhancers)
- Vegan patties and sausages (contain additives, flavor enhancers, and salicylates)

Eczema-Healthy Protein Sources

- Turkey
- Beans, canned or dried beans (except fava beans)
- Beans, green
- Lamb
- Lentil sprouts
- Lentils
- Mung bean sprouts
- Salmon or tuna canned in springwater or brine
- Trout, rainbow trout
- Veal
- White fish, fresh
- Preservative-free ground lamb, chicken, veal

How Much Protein?

Ensure you consume some sort of protein every day — preferably in two of your main meals. Between $1\frac{1}{2}$ oz (45 g) and $3\frac{1}{2}$ oz (100 g) of cooked meat will provide adults with sufficient daily protein, as will two small lean lamb chops, two slices of roast beef, or half a chicken breast. A $2\frac{1}{2}$- to $4\frac{1}{2}$-oz (80 to 120 g) serving of fish will also give you enough protein for the day.

If you're vegetarian or vegan, eat 2 servings of vegetarian protein every day (children and pregnant women should have 2 or 3 servings) alongside a grain, such as brown rice. This makes the protein more "complete." One cup (250 mL) of lentils, green beans, chickpeas, split peas, or kidney beans served with whole-grain carbohydrates will provide your daily protein needs.

19. Legumes

Legumes are rich in magnesium and potassium and supply dietary fiber, protein, and slow-release carbohydrates for energy. Canned legumes, such as brown lentils, chickpeas, and mixed beans, are a convenient option. However, some nutrients are destroyed during the canning process and some cans are coated with bisphenol A (BPA), which can leach into the canned food. The Food Standards Agency in the United Kingdom says that BPA is known to have "weak estrogenic effects" and it could disrupt hormone systems, although more research is warranted. If using canned legumes, it is also essential to drain and thoroughly rinse them because they are packed with a fair amount of salt. Dried legumes that are home-cooked are the best and most nutritious choice.

Guidelines for Cooking Legumes

Step 1: Rinsing and sorting

Whether using canned or dried legumes, rinse the legumes and pick out any discolored or shriveled legumes or small stones.

Step 2: Soaking dried legumes

Most dried legumes should be soaked overnight in water. This helps to reduce phytic acid, to promote even cooking, and to reduce simmering time. For every 1 cup (250 mL) of legumes, use 4 cups (1 L) of water.

Long-soak method: Place legumes and water in a saucepan, cover, and soak overnight at room temperature (at least 8 hours). In the morning, discard the water and use new water for cooking.

Quick-soak method: Boil the legumes in water for 5 minutes and then remove from heat, cover, and soak for 2 hours. Discard the water. Then add fresh water for cooking (refer to Step 3).

If you have flatulence problems when eating beans, combine both methods: bring a large saucepan of water to boil, then add the legumes and boil for 2 minutes. Remove from heat, cover, and soak overnight. Important: discard the soaked water because it contains the indigestible sugars that promote gas.

Step 3: Cooking legumes

After soaking the legumes (if required), add the necessary amount of water. Avoid stirring the beans while cooking because it can damage them. Do not add salt because it can toughen the beans if added too early.

Lentils are quick to cook, but for all other beans, check their progress after 45 minutes using this simple test: if the legumes are cooked, they should be soft enough to easily mash using the back of a fork. All cooking times are approximate and will vary depending on how long it has been since they were harvested.

Did You Know?

No Soaking

Dried lentils (red and brown/green), split peas (green and yellow), and black-eyed peas do not need to be soaked. Adzuki and mung beans only need to be soaked for 1 to 2 hours. However, make sure you rinse these beans and lentils thoroughly, changing the water two or three times until it runs clear.

Cooking Times for Legumes

Legume Variety	Approximate Cooking Time
Adzuki	45 minutes to 1½ hours
Black-eyed peas/beans	1 to 2 hours
Cannellini beans	1 hour
Chickpeas	1½ to 2 hours (allow to cool in cooking water)
Dried split peas	Up to 45 minutes
Kidney beans	1 hour or more
Lentils	20 to 30 minutes
Lima beans	1 to 2 hours
Mung beans	45 to 60 minutes
Navy beans	1 to 2 hours
Pinto beans	1 to 2 hours

20. Sea Salt

Commercial table salt is not eczema-safe because it can include an added anti-caking agent containing aluminum, because most of the nutritious minerals have been removed, and because it's acid-producing, so it can disrupt the body's acid-alkaline balance. If you'd like to use salt, buy quality Celtic or natural sea salt — eczema-safe salt should be gray in color, indicating it's unprocessed and mineral-rich, and it should not contain an anti-caking agent. These alkaline salts are okay to use in moderation. Do not add salt to your food if you have high blood pressure.

Diet Status Questionnaire

This questionnaire is designed to determine your nutritional status before starting the Eczema Diet. The questions are suitable for adults and children with eczema, and if you have a baby with eczema, you can use this questionnaire to assess maternal diet (the diet of the mother during pregnancy and breastfeeding or the diet of both parents before conception). Use a checkmark to highlight the answer that best suits your experience (yes = weekly or daily; sometimes = monthly or occasionally; no = never or rarely; unsure = not known).

EATING HABITS	Yes	Sometimes	No	Unsure
Do you eat or drink any of the following or experience these reactions?				
Part 1: Egg Whites (Egg White Injury)				
Eat raw egg or raw egg whites				
Consume whole-egg mayonnaise				
Eat mayonnaise, coleslaw, or creamy salad dressings				
Drink protein shakes containing powdered/fresh egg or egg whites				
Eat the icing on traditional wedding cakes				
Experience mood disturbances, such as depression, moodiness, or anxiety				
Eat traditional chocolate mousse (store-bought varieties may not contain egg, but they have lots of artificial additives)				
Have dermatitis plus any of the following symptoms: grayish pallor of the skin, scaly lips, nausea, loss of appetite, muscle pain, raised cholesterol, or localized numbness				
Eat store-bought dips containing egg				
Part 2: Vegetable Oils				
Use margarine				
Use canola oil, plain vegetable oil, olive oil, or "light" cooking oil				
Consume store-bought pastry or softened butter (containing vegetable oil and additives)				
Eat fried foods (e.g., fish and chips or takeout foods cooked in oil)				
Part 3: Salicylates				
Eat a lot of fruit (3 servings/1½ cups/375 mL or more daily)				
Frequently eat fava beans, broccoli, cauliflower, eggplant, gherkins, olives, mushrooms, Swiss chard, or spinach				

EATING HABITS	Yes	Sometimes	No	Unsure
Frequently eat tomatoes, oranges, lemon, kiwifruit, or strawberries				
Drink tea, herbal tea, or coffee				
Drink tomato juice, flavored sodas, or cordial				
Part 4: MSG and Flavor Enhancers				
Drink beer, wine, hard cider, brandy, liqueur, port, rum, or sherry				
Eat corn flakes cereal or consume corn products				
Have adverse reactions to aspirin				
Part 5: Part 5: Artificial Chemicals (General)				
Eat dried prunes, raisins, sultanas, tomato and/or tomato products, such as pizza sauces and juice				
Eat broccoli, mushrooms, Swiss chard, or spinach				
Eat deli meats, such as turkey, chicken, salami, and sausages				
Consume gravy, soy sauce, flavored potato chips, or flavored rice crackers				
Part 6. Personal Hygiene and Treats				
Chew gum or use mouthwash				
Eat candy				

Score: Let's take a look at the results to identify where you might need to alter your diet.

Part 1: Egg Whites (Egg White Injury)
Assess your total intake of raw egg whites. If you consume whole-egg mayonnaise once a week and tuna dip once a week, this is classified as frequent consumption of raw egg white. Egg white injury may result. (For egg white injury and biotin information, see "Egg White Injury and Biotin," page 100.)

Part 2: Vegetable Oils
If you consume margarine, products containing margarine, or vegetable oils, discontinue use and refer to "Rice Bran Oil" (page 72).

Part 3: Salicylates
This section highlights foods and drinks rich in salicylates. Do not consume these products while on the Eczema Diet because doing so may affect your results. (If you have been prescribed aspirin for heart disease, do not stop taking aspirin, but talk to your doctor about your options.)

Part 4: MSG and Flavor Enhancers
This section highlights foods and drinks rich in natural MSG and foods containing artificial flavor enhancers. Do not consume these products while on the Eczema Diet because doing so may affect your results.

Part 5: Artificial Chemicals (General)
Do not consume these products while on the Eczema Diet.

Part 6: Personal Hygiene and Treats
Avoid these products while on the Eczema Diet.

Chapter 4

Eczema-Healthy Food Guides

The food charts in this chapter are designed to show you what foods to favor and what foods to avoid or limit if you have eczema. Selecting eczema-healthy foods takes some practice as you assess their various properties — their acidity and alkalinity, their ratio of omega-3 to omega-6, their salicylate and raw egg white content, to name a few. To assist you in choosing eczema-healthy foods, we have created a set of food guides you can use in planning meals, shopping for ingredients, and preparing the recipes.

At first, these food lists seem restrictive, but as you work your way through the Eczema Diet program, you add more and more food items to the eczema-safe and eczema-healthy list. By the time you reach Stage 3, you will have all the safe and healthy foods you need to prepare the recipes in this book.

Q. How much protein should I eat at lunch and dinner — for that matter, how many vegetables and breads?

A. A simple rule when serving lunch and dinner is this: fill half your plate with vegetables, one-quarter with quality protein (meat, fish, beans), and the other quarter with quality carbohydrates (rice, quinoa, spelt bread). If you want dessert, favor eczema-safe fruits, such as banana, papaya, or pear. These rules also apply to children; just use appropriate child-sized plates and read protein information on portion sizes. For more information on serving a balanced diet, read the United States Department of Agriculture (USDA) guide to good nutrition, called MyPlate, and Eating Well with Canada's Food Guide, published by Health Canada.

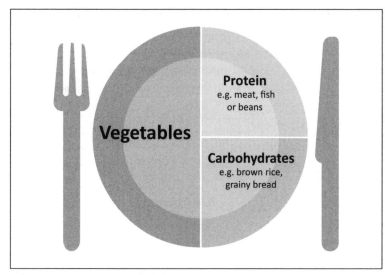

Alternatives and Substitutions

This handy table distills the advice given in the last chapter (on foods to avoid) and presents convenient alternatives and substitutions that can help to heal your eczema. This information applies directly to Stage 1 of the Eczema Diet program. To compile a shopping list, check off the food items in the "Eczema-Healthy Alternatives and Recipes" column and record the ingredients from the recipes identified in the recipe section of this book. There is no need to buy all of these ingredients during one shopping trip. Buy a few each time you shop.

Alternatives and Substitutions

Foods to Avoid	Food Group	Eczema-Healthy Alternatives and Recipes
Milk, cheese, butter, yogurt (made from cow's, goat's, and sheep's milk)	Dairy Products	Dairy substitutes, organic rice milk, oat milk, plus organic soy milk in moderation (not containing "soy isolate")
Margarine, dairy-free margarine, softened butter	Oils and Fats	Sesame-Free Hummus (page 239) Bean Dip (page 240) Banana Carob Spread (page 238) (Stage 2: pure organic butter or ghee if no allergy to dairy)
Pork, ham, bacon, beef, deli meats, sausages, ground meats with preservatives	Meat and Meat Products	Lean lamb, organic chicken, beef bones used in broth, lean ground lamb/veal/chicken (ask butcher for additive-free or freshly ground meats)
Smoked salmon and other smoked fish, canned tuna in oil or olive oil	Fish and Fish Products	Baked or grilled trout or smaller white fish
Egg, raw white, whole-egg mayonnaise, dips with egg	Eggs	Egg replacements (baking section) Sesame-Free Hummus (page 239) instead of mayonnaise (Stage 2: free-range egg, cooked, 1 to 2 eggs a week maximum, if not allergic to egg)
Most fruits, fruit juices	Fruit	Peeled pear, banana (not sugar variety), papaya
Tomato, tomato-containing products, bell pepper, mushrooms, pumpkin, broccoli	Vegetables	Carrot, celery, potato, sweet potato, green beans, Brussels sprouts, cabbage (white and red)
Dark leafy greens, spinach, Swiss chard, arugula (in Stage 1 of diet)	Vegetables	Romaine lettuce, iceberg lettuce
Most herbs and spices (in Stage 1 of diet)	Flavorings	Fresh parsley (in moderation), parsley flakes, chives
Onions, most sprouts	Vegetables	Leeks, green onions, garlic, dried garlic powder, mung bean sprouts, lentil sprouts, sprouted spelt
Soy sauce, tamari, salad dressings of any kind, ketchup, barbecue sauce, and other sauces	Flavorings	Sesame-Free Hummus (page 239) Parsley Pesto (page 241) Omega Salad Dressing (page 220) (Stage 2 only)
Avocado	Fruit	Sesame-Free Hummus (page 239) Bean Dip (page 240)

Foods to Avoid	Food Group	Eczema-Healthy Alternatives and Recipes
Dried fruits	Fruit	Peeled pear, papaya, banana Baked Banana Chips (page 242)
Nuts	Nuts and Seeds	Unsalted raw cashews (if no allergy to nuts; do not have roasted)
Vinegar (all types), pickled foods	Preservatives and Flavoring	(Stage 2 only: quality apple cider vinegar, if no allergy to sulfites)
Olive oil, canola oil, coconut oil, vegetable oils	Cooking Oils	Rice bran oil
Wheat products, wheat flour, white flour, wheat bread, commercial wheat breakfast cereals, wheat pasta	Grains and Flour Products	Spelt flour, spelt sourdough, buckwheat, brown rice, basmati rice, quinoa, whole or rolled oats, rice bran, brown rice flour, white rice flour, barley, rye, potato flour, soy flour, rye flour, plain gluten-free bread (no corn or cornmeal), gluten-free rice pasta, buckwheat pasta
Corn, corn flakes cereal, corn chips	Grains, corn	Quinoa porridge, rolled oat porridge, puffed rice cereal (preferably brown), occasional use of white cornstarch (e.g., in gluten-free baking) is acceptable, plain rice crackers (no additives)
Fava beans	Legumes	Kidney beans, navy beans, lentils, cannellini beans, chickpeas, green beans
Sugar, honey, molasses, artificial sweeteners, cocoa powder	Sweeteners	Rice malt syrup, pure maple syrup, golden syrup (used only in baking), carob powder, pure vanilla extract
Soft drinks, diet soft drinks, flavored mineral water	Beverages	Filtered water, natural springwater (not carbonated)
Coffee, tea, herbal tea (all kinds)	Beverages	Therapeutic Broth (page 212) Tarzan Juice (page 207) Healthy Skin Juice (page 206) Healthy Skin Smoothie (page 209) Chocolate Milk (page 210)
Tap water		Filtered water, natural springwater (not carbonated)
Biscuits, cookies, muffins, snack foods, cakes, pastries, chips, pancake mix, confectionery, lollipops, candy, chocolate, jams, spreads	Grains, baked goods	Carrot and celery sticks Pear Muffins (page 203) Spelt Pancakes (page 201) Buckwheat Crêpes (page 202) Plain rice crackers/cakes (no additives) with Banana Carob Spread (page 238) Baked Banana Chips (page 242) New Anzac Cookies (page 250) (occasional consumption only)

Eczema-Healthy Foods Classified by Food Group

The food items in this table are divided into Stage 1 and Stage 2 of the Eczema Diet program and are classified by food group, much like the USDA does in the MyPlate food guide. Stage 1 lists the main food products to buy while you have eczema, and the Stage 2 guide should be used after your eczema clears up.

These shopping lists do not account for age and feeding ability, and not all ingredients are suitable for small children or those with gluten intolerance (or less common allergies, such as rice allergy). The shopping lists include ingredients that are not in the Eczema Diet recipes, so you have the option to use them to make your own recipes. This can be useful if you have food allergies to some of the foods in Stage 1 and you need alternatives to increase variety in your diet. Do not try to buy every food item on this list immediately. Instead, work your way toward recovery item by item.

Brands

Beware of differences in brands. For example, the flavor, texture, and general suitability of gluten-free products, such as pasta, can vary considerably between brands, so if you don't like one or find your skin is not improving as it should on the diet, please persevere and try others until you discover the ones that work for you.

Further Information

For a more comprehensive guide to eczema-safe foods, see the charts in Part 6: Planning the Eczema Diet (pages 174–182). The pH and the salicylates, sulfites, amines, glycemic index, and gluten content of common foods are analyzed.

Stage 1 and Stage 2 Safe Foods Guide

Food Group	Stage 1 Food Items	Stage 2 Food Items
Fruits	Bananas (not sugar variety), Papaya, Pears	Apples, golden delicious, Apples, red delicious, Bananas, Blueberries, Lemon, Lime, Papaya, Pears, Watermelon
Vegetables & Herbs	Beets, fresh, Brussels sprouts, Cabbage, red or white, Carrots, Celery, Chives (not in recipes), Garlic (not Chinese), Green beans, Green onions, Leeks, Lettuce, iceberg, Lettuce, romaine, Mung bean sprouts (fresh only/check use-by date), Parsley, Potatoes, new, Rutabaga, Sweet potato	Asparagus, Baby (pattypan) squash, Bamboo shoots (not in recipes), Basil, Beets, fresh, Bok choy, Brussels sprouts, Cabbage, red or white, Carrots, Celery, Chicory, Chives, Cilantro, fresh, Endive, Garlic (not Chinese), Green beans, Green onions, Green peas, Ketchup, organic, Lettuce, iceberg, Lettuce, romaine, Mint, Mung bean sprouts, Onion, red or white, Parsley, Potatoes (white), Snow pea shoots, Snow peas, Sweet potato, Turnip, Yam
Grains, breads, & cereals	Barley, Buckwheat pasta (wheat-free), Buckwheat, roasted (not in recipes), Gluten-free bread, if necessary (preservative-free; check ingredients), Gluten-free pasta (preferable to pastas that are not gluten-free, Rice, basmati (not jasmine or other white rice), Rice, brown (not quick/instant rice), Spelt sourdough bread (preservative-free)	Barley, Buckwheat pasta (wheat-free), Buckwheat, roasted (not in recipes), Gluten-free bread, if necessary (preservative-free; check ingredients), Gluten-free pasta, Puffed brown rice cereal, plain, Quinoa grains (not puffed), Rice, basmati, Rice, brown, Rolled oats (wheat-free if possible), Spelt sourdough bread (preservative-free)
Crackers & biscuits	Puffed brown rice cereal, plain (not in recipes), Quinoa grains (not puffed), Rolled oats (preferably wheat-free), Rye crispbread, whole wheat, Whole-grain or plain rice crackers (no flavor enhancers), Whole-grain plain rice cakes (no flavor enhancers or corn)	Rye crispbread, whole wheat, Whole-grain or plain rice crackers (no flavor enhancers), Whole-grain plain rice cakes (no flavor enhancers, no corn)
Baking & flours	Arrowroot flour (not in recipes), Baking powder (for baking; not in recipes), Baking soda (for baking), Buckwheat flour, Citric acid (flavor/lemon replacer; found in baking section), Egg replacer/substitute, Gluten-free self-rising flour, Rice flour (preferably brown), Rye flour (not in recipes), Soy flour (not in recipes), Spelt flour (preferably whole-grain)	Arrowroot flour (not in recipes), Baking powder (for baking; not in recipes), Baking soda (for baking), Buckwheat flour, Citric acid (flavor/lemon replacer; found in baking section), Egg replacer/substitute, Gluten-free self-rising flour, Rice flour (preferably brown), Rye flour (not in recipes), Soy flour (not in recipes), Spelt flour

Stage 1 and Stage 2 Safe Foods Guide *(continued)*

Food Group	Stage 1 Food Items	Stage 2 Food Items
Meat & Fish	*(Note: do not buy all items on the same day)* Chicken: 1 large or 2 small chicken carcasses for Therapeutic Broth recipe (page 212) Beef: 2 large beef bones with a little meat on them for Therapeutic Broth recipe Chicken: free-range/organic, antibiotic-free (thigh fillets, breast, or whole for roasting) Lamb: frenched cutlets or lean lamb, fat trimmed Fish: sardines, salmon canned in springwater or brine (no flavorings or oil), trout, rainbow trout (not frozen or preserved/packaged) Tuna: quality tuna, chunky, canned in springwater or brine (not oil or olive oil) Turkey: uncooked or organic (not deli slices; no flavor enhancer; not in recipes) Veal: lean (e.g., veal steaks; not pre-crumbed; not in recipes)	*(Note: do not buy all items on the same day)* Chicken: free range/organic, antibiotic-free (thigh fillets, breast, or whole for roasting); use 2 chicken carcasses for Therapeutic Broth recipe (page 212); or chicken necks, lamb/beef bones Eggs: free-range eggs or egg substitute Catfish or small white fish (not basa, snapper, swordfish, marlin, perch, or tuna) Lamb: lean lamb (not shanks or cheap ground) Salmon (not frozen or preserved/packaged) Salmon: canned in springwater or brine (no flavorings or oil) Trout, rainbow trout (not frozen or preserved/packaged) Tuna: quality tuna, chunky, canned in springwater or brine (not oil or olive oil) Turkey: uncooked or organic (not deli slices; no flavor enhancers) Firm tofu, plain/unflavored (optional, not tempeh or vegan patties) Veal: lean (e.g., veal steaks; not pre-crumbed; not in recipes)
Non-Dairy Milk & Drinks	Malt-free soy milk option, Oat milk, Organic rice milk option, Organic soy milk (favor refrigerated over long-life tetra; favor organic whole soybean milk, not soy isolate; no flavorings)	Malt-free soy milk option, Oat milk, Organic rice milk option, Organic soy milk
Legumes, Beans, Seeds, & Nuts	Beans, dried (kidney, cannellini, etc.; not fava beans), Canned beans, Cashew nuts, raw, unsalted, Chickpeas, dried or canned, Red lentils, dried, Soy lecithin granules, Soybeans, fresh or dried (not in recipes), Split peas, dried (not in recipes)	Beans, dried (kidney, cannellini, etc.; not fava beans), Brown lentils, canned, Canned beans (no flavorings), Cashew nuts, raw, unsalted, Chickpeas, dried or canned, Red lentils, dried, Soy lecithin granules, Soybeans, fresh or dried (not in recipes), Split peas, dried (green or yellow) (not in recipes)

Stage 1 and Stage 2 Safe Foods Guide *(continued)*

Food Group	Stage 1 Food Items	Stage 2 Food Items
Oils & Fats	Flaxseed oil (must be refrigerated; preferably organic), Flax seeds, whole (not pre-ground; not a ground mixture of flax, sunflower, and almond, or LSA), Rice bran oil	Apple cider vinegar (organic; not "double strength"), Flaxseed oil (must be refrigerated; preferably organic), Flax seeds, whole, Pure organic butter (allergy permitting; no additives or oils)
Sweeteners & Flavorings	Carob powder (not cocoa powder), Celtic sea salt or natural sea salt (no anti-caking agent), Dried garlic powder (no additives; not garlic salt), Dried parsley flakes, Golden syrup (if baking), Pure maple syrup (optional), Rice malt syrup, Vanilla bean or pure vanilla extract	Carob powder (not cocoa powder), Celtic sea salt or natural sea salt (no anti-caking agent), Cinnamon, Dried garlic powder (no additives; not garlic salt), Dried parsley flakes, Golden syrup (if baking), Ground cumin, Pure maple syrup (optional), Rice malt syrup, Vanilla bean or pure vanilla extract
Favorites (add your own favorite items to the list!)		

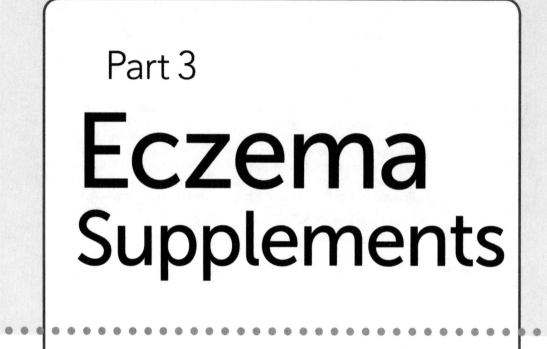

Part 3

Eczema
Supplements

Chapter 5
Top 15 Nutrient Supplements

If you have eczema, your food may not be rich enough in several nutrients to promote healing. In these cases, you will need to take supplements. These nutrients work together to repair, renew, and moisturize your skin. Use these supplements in conjunction with eczema-healthy foods, but not with any herbal preparations containing vegetable extracts, such as broccoli, which are rich in salicylates and other plant chemicals. You don't want to inadvertently increase your chemical burden. Some nutrients work synergistically with others.

1. Vitamin C

The body is truly remarkable and resourceful. It makes many of its own vitamins in the gastrointestinal tract and it stores minerals in the liver and bones; however, the body does not store or manufacture vitamin C, so it must be consumed in your diet. Vitamin C (also known as ascorbic acid) aids the absorption of iron and copper, is vital for the formation of collagen in the skin, guards against infections, and is required for liver detoxification. Vitamin C is a natural antihistamine, destroying the imidazole ring of the histamine molecule. For this reason, it is imperative that eczema sufferers avoid developing vitamin C deficiency because it can result in histamine toxicity and allergic reactions may increase in severity. You can prevent this from occurring by eating vitamin C–rich papaya or Brussels sprouts, and by taking a vitamin C supplement. To meet your daily requirement for vitamin C (in amounts that are adequate for preventing histamine toxicity), vitamin C–rich fruits and vegetables must be eaten daily. For example, eat sliced papaya on porridge in the morning, in a side salad with lunch, and with green beans and Brussels sprouts with dinner.

> According to some recent research, Americans continue to suffer from scurvy (the "sailor's disease" of the 1700s) because people aren't eating enough fruit and vegetables.

Vitamin C Deficiency

Signs of vitamin C deficiency include allergies, dry skin, bumpy/rough skin, easy bruising, small purplish spots on skin, fatigue, depression, tooth loss, hemorrhaging, bleeding gums, swelling of lower extremities, joint pain (mimics arthritis), and poor wound healing. In infants, low or no intake of vitamin C from breast milk when the mother is vitamin C deficient can mimic shaken baby syndrome (easy bruising, brain hemorrhage, blood pooling in the eyes, and fractures). According to some recent research, Americans continue to suffer from scurvy (the "sailor's disease" of the 1700s) because people aren't eating enough fruit and vegetables.

Vitamin C deficiency can occur from dieting, vaccinations/immunizations, frequent aspirin intake, high salicylate ingestion, the birth control pill, stress, cigarette smoking, diabetes, or following a no-fruit diet (such as high-protein, low-carb diets). Not all fruits and vegetables contain adequate vitamin C.

Common Food Sources of Vitamin C

Food Source	Serving	Vitamin C Content
Guava (not suitable during Stage 1)	3½ oz (100 g)	245 mg
Brussels sprouts	3½ oz (100 g)	110 mg
Papaya	5 oz (150 g)	90 mg
Cabbage	3½ oz (100 g)	45 mg
Leek	3½ oz (100 g)	30 mg
Potato	1 medium	30 mg
Rutabaga, turnip	3½ oz (100 g)	25 mg
Sweet potato	3½ oz (100 g)	25 mg
Green beans	3½ oz (100 g)	20 mg
Banana	1 medium	15 mg
Green onions	3	15 mg
Parsley	⅓ oz (10 g)	10 mg

Total Daily Intake of Vitamin C (Ascorbic Acid)

Age Range	Total Daily Intake	Dosing
Adults	200–500 mg	60 mg twice daily in supplement form, taken with food; consume 2½ cups (625 mL) fruits and vegetables daily, supplying approximately 200 mg vitamin C
5–17 years	70–120 mg	30 mg twice daily in supplement form, taken with food; consume 1½ cups (375 mL) fruits and vegetables
1–4 years	60–100 mg	15 mg twice daily in supplement form, taken with food; consume 1 cup (250 mL) fruits and vegetables
0–12 months	25–35 mg	Vitamin C is sourced from breast milk or formula; also give infants on solids 1 tablespoon to ½ cup (15 to 125 mL) of fruits and vegetables daily, depending on age and appetite

Caution

Do not chew vitamin C tablets, because they can wear away teeth enamel, making teeth sensitive and painful. A powdered multi-formula supplement is preferable (especially for children, to avoid choking), or a solid tablet swallowed whole.

Vitamin C thins the blood. If nose bleeding occurs, halve the vitamin C dosage or take vitamin K at the same time. Do not take vitamin C supplements if you have hemochromatosis or if you have been prescribed aspirin, anticoagulants, or antidepressants.

Powerful Co-Nutrients

The benefits of vitamin C can increase when taken with other nutrients.

- Vitamin C + vitamin B3
- Vitamin C + glycine (collagen formation and liver detoxification)
- Vitamin C + quercetin + vitamin B6 (natural antihistamines)

2. Glycine

Glycine is an amino acid found in protein that is beneficial for eczema sufferers for many reasons: it is anti-inflammatory, cell protective, and vital for collagen synthesis in the skin. Collagen is the glue that binds the skin together, making it strong and attractive. Approximately one-third of collagen is composed of glycine. Glycine plays a role in the liver's detoxification of chemicals, and supplementation can significantly reduce salicylate sensitivity. Glycine helps to heal the damaged skin barrier.

Glycine is classed as a "non-essential" amino acid because the body is supposed to be able to manufacture its own supply if your diet is good. However, in eczema sufferers, the ability to manufacturer glycine may not be adequate and/or the glycine receptors in their skin may be compromised. According to researchers from the University of Heidelberg in Germany, people with eczema and psoriasis have a striking reduction in glycine receptors in the skin.

Dosage Notes: See a physician or dietitian before giving your baby glycine. Take powdered glycine mixed with water before meals. After your eczema clears up, gradually cut down on the supplement dosage to half the dosage or less.

Common Food Sources of Glycine

Food Source	Serving	Glycine Content
Broth	Therapeutic Broth recipe (page 212)	Glycine content varies
Flax seeds	⅔ oz (20 g)	250 mg
Gelatin, unsweetened dry powder	⅓ oz (10 g)	1904 mg
Soybeans	3½ oz (100 g)	1880 mg
Quail	3½ oz (100 g)	1542 mg
Turkey or chicken, with skin	3½ oz (100 g)	1395 mg
Split peas, raw	3½ oz (100 g)	1092 mg
Blue crab meat	3½ oz (100 g)	1089 mg
Veal, raw	3½ oz (100 g)	1078 mg
Tuna, raw	3½ oz (100 g)	1056 mg
Buckwheat	3½ oz (100 g)	1031 mg
Salmon, raw	3½ oz (100 g)	1022 mg
Red lentils, raw	3½ oz (100 g)	1014 mg
Rainbow trout, raw	3½ oz (100 g)	1002 mg

Total Daily Intake of Glycine

Age Range	Total Daily Intake	Dosing
Adults	2000–3000 mg	1000 mg daily in supplement form
13–18 years	800–1000 mg	500 mg daily in supplement form
5–12 years	600–800 mg	250–300 mg daily in supplement form
0–12 months		Breastfeeding mothers can take glycine to increase glycine in breast milk; glycine is in infant formulas but not in adequate amounts; speak to your health-care provider

Caution

High-dose glycine taken over long periods of more than 6 months can cause muscle aches at night if you are low in estrogen. If this occurs, discontinue use. Do not take glycine if you are on blood-thinning medications, such as aspirin, because glycine will reduce the effects of aspirin (it literally detoxifies it). If you are taking medications, seek medical advice before taking liver detoxification supplements.

Powerful Co-Nutrients

The benefits of glycine can increase when taken with other nutrients.

- Glycine + magnesium + vitamin B6 (liver detoxification/glycination pathway)

- Glycine + cysteine + glutamine (for glutathione) + vitamin B2 + vitamin B6 + vitamin C + Brussels sprouts or cabbage (for liver detoxification in the glutathionation pathway)

3. Biotin

Biotin is a B vitamin (vitamin B7) found in egg whites. Eating too much raw egg white can aggravate eczema symptoms, causing egg white injury, but biotin can balance this situation. Raw egg whites are found in dips, whole-egg mayonnaise, and coleslaw dressing. Some health experts recommend protein shakes containing fresh or powdered egg whites. We lick the bowl when making cakes or pancake mix containing raw egg. Traditional chocolate mousse and wedding cake icing contain raw egg whites. It may not be a coincidence that egg allergy is the number one allergy with which eczema sufferers present (and often they are only allergic to raw eggs).

Eating raw egg whites on the rare occasion won't cause problems — egg white injury is achieved if you frequently eat dips, creamy dressings, whole-egg mayonnaise, and other sources of raw egg whites.

Did You Know?

Egg White Injury and Biotin

In 1942, scientists first demonstrated the need for biotin in the diet. They induced "egg white injury," where the consumption of avidin, a protein in raw egg whites, latches onto the B-group vitamin called biotin so your body cannot use it. Biotin is required for delta-6-desaturase enzyme reactions in the body, and when this enzyme malfunctions from lack of biotin, skin inflammation is the first sign to appear. Biotin deficiency symptoms are dermatitis or eczema, grayish pallor of the skin, scaly lips, nausea, loss of appetite, depression, moodiness, muscle pain, raised cholesterol, and localized numbness.

Common Food Sources of Biotin

Food Source	Serving	Biotin Content
Chicken liver*	3½ oz (100 g)	170 mcg
Soybeans, cooked	1 cup	40 mcg
Oysters	12	18 mcg
Egg	1	15 mcg
Salmon, grilled	5 oz (150 g)	14 mcg
Rolled (porridge) oats	2 oz (60 g)	12 mcg
Tuna, canned	3½ oz (100 g)	3 mcg

*Caution: Liver is the organ that stores and processes chemicals, hormones and pesticides, so do not consume liver unless it is organic.

Total Daily Intake of Biotin

Age Range	Total Daily Intake	Dosing
Adults	100–150 mcg	Supplement form
5–17 years	50–75 mcg	Supplement form
1–4 years	10–50 mcg	Supplement form
0–12 months		Obtain biotin through breast milk or infant formula, or speak to a nutritionist about biotin supplementation

Biotin can be manufactured by friendly bacteria in healthy intestines, but this may not occur in rash-prone individuals due to genetics, high omega-6 intake, antibiotic use, a bout of diarrhea, or illness. The biotin in food is usually attached to protein and is poorly absorbed by the body, so a biotin supplement is essential for eczema sufferers.

Caution

High-dose biotin supplementation may lessen the effect of some cholesterol medications.

Powerful Synergistic Co-Nutrients

The benefits of biotin can increase when taken with other nutrients.
- Biotin + vitamin B6 + magnesium + zinc (for delta-6-desaturase enzyme reactions)

4. Vitamin B$_6$

Vitamin B$_6$ (also known as pyridoxine) is involved in more than 100 enzyme reactions, including delta-6-desaturase, which helps to reduce inflammation. Vitamin B$_6$ is essential for eczema and allergy sufferers because it's a natural antihistamine and it helps to reduce salicylate and monosodium glutamate (MSG) sensitivity. Vitamin B$_6$ deficiency signs include dermatitis, irritability, mood changes, convulsions, numbness or cramps in the arms and legs, anemia, smooth, painful tongue, ulcers inside the mouth, skin cracks at the corners of the mouth or eyes, low blood sugar/hypoglycemia, and poor immunity (decreased lymphocytes and interleukin-2). Vitamin B$_6$ deficiency can be caused by or is associated with frequent alcohol consumption, poor diet, a high-protein diet (this increases the need for vitamin B$_6$), prescription drugs (such as anticonvulsants, antiturberculosis, and penicillamine), cirrhosis of the liver, and malabsorption syndromes.

Caution

If you are taking prescription medications, speak to a nutritionist or doctor before taking a vitamin B$_6$ supplement.

Powerful Co-Nutrients

The benefits of vitamin B$_6$ can increase when taken with other nutrients.

- Vitamin B$_6$ + biotin + magnesium + zinc (anti-inflammatory delta-6-desaturase enzymes)
- Vitamin B$_6$ + glycine + magnesium (glycination, Phase 2 liver detoxification)

Common Food Sources of Vitamin B6

Food Source	Serving	Vitamin B6 Content
Salmon, grilled	5 oz (150 g)	1.20 mg
Muesli (granola)	2 oz (60 g)	0.96 mg
Bran cereal	1½ oz (40 g)	0.75 mg
Potato	1 medium	0.70 mg
Wheat germ	2 tbsp (20 mL)	0.66 mg
Tuna, canned	3½ oz (100 g)	0.50 mg
Lentils, cooked	1 cup (250 mL)	0.45 mg
Beef, cooked	5 oz (150 g)	0.44 mg
Chicken or turkey, cooked	5 oz (150 g)	0.40 mg
Brussels sprouts	3½ oz (100 g)	0.37 mg
Banana	1 medium	0.35 mg
Buckwheat	2½ oz (75 g)	0.32 mg
Rolled (porridge) oats	2 oz (60 g)	0.19 mg
Cashews	1 oz (30 g)	0.16 mg

Total Daily Intake of Vitamin B6

Age Range	Total Daily Intake	Dosing
Adults	8–13 mg	Supplement form
5–17 years	4 mg	Supplement form
1–4 years	1–2 mg	Supplement form
0–12 months	0.5 mg	Obtain vitamin B6 through breast milk or infant formula

5. Magnesium

Magnesium is an alkaline mineral known as "the great relaxer" because it relieves muscle tension and stiffness, and it can decrease cravings for alcohol. Magnesium is needed for the functioning of more than 300 enzymes in the human body, it helps to alkalize the blood, and it decreases chemical sensitivity when combined with glycine and vitamin B6. Magnesium deficiency can be caused by diarrhea, poor diet, a low-protein diet (less than 1 oz/30 g daily), fat malabsorption, frequent alcohol consumption, and the frequent use of antibiotics or diuretics. Magnesium absorption declines as you age.

Caution

Magnesium supplementation can interfere with digoxin (heart medicine), some antibiotics, chlorpromazine (tranquilizer), penicillamine, oral anticoagulants, and some antimalaria drugs. Do not take magnesium at the same time as drugs to treat osteoporosis (take them at least 2 hours apart).

Powerful Co-Nutrients

The benefits of magnesium can increase when taken with other nutrients.

- Magnesium + vitamin B6 + biotin + zinc (for delta-6-desaturase enzyme)
- Magnesium + vitamin B6 + glycine (glycination, Phase 2 liver detoxification)

6. Zinc

Zinc is vital for skin repair and maintenance. Deficiency leads to skin lesions, dry and rough skin, and delayed wound healing. A severe zinc deficiency, caused by faulty gene expression, induces bullous pustular dermatitis (blister-like dermatitis), patches of eczema, and hair loss (alopecia). Other deficiency signs include acne, stretch marks, white-coated tongue, white spots on fingernails, impotence, infertility, frequent infections, frizzy hair, poor sense of taste or smell, and premature aging of the skin. During your teenage years, zinc is needed for rapid growth spurts. The skin's oil-gland activity is regulated by zinc, and deficiency can lead to acne.

> Zinc is vital for skin repair and maintenance. Deficiency leads to skin lesions, dry and rough skin, and delayed wound healing.

Common Food Sources of Magnesium

Food Source	Serving	Magnesium Content
Bran cereal	1½ oz (40 g)	115 mg
Rolled oats	2 oz (60 g)	80 mg
Brown rice, cooked	1 cup (250 mL)	80 mg
Dried beans, cooked	1 cup (250 mL)	75 mg
Wheat germ	2 tbsp (30 mL)	65 mg
Shrimp	3½ oz (100 g)	60 mg
Canned sardines	3½ oz (100 g)	60 mg
Oysters	12	60 mg
Fish	Average serving	50 mg
Chicken or red meat	Average serving	30 mg
Whole wheat bread	2 slices	40 mg
White bread	2 slices	15 mg

Total Daily Intake of Magnesium

Age Range	Total Daily Intake	Dosing
Adults	350–400 mg	20–60 mg in supplement form; the rest should be supplied by a healthy diet
5–17 years	240–350 mg	10 mg in supplement form; the rest should be supplied by a healthy diet
1–4 years	130 mg	5–10 mg in supplement form; the rest should be supplied by a healthy diet
0–12 months	30–75 mg	Obtain magnesium through breast milk or infant formula

Menstruation and ejaculation deplete zinc stores in the body. Zinc deficiency can be caused by frequent alcohol consumption, high salt intake (from canned food, takeout, and restaurant food), high calcium intake, chronic stress, frequent consumption of coffee or tea, and high-fiber diets rich in phytic acid (which is why soaking grains is recommended, see "Soaking Grains," page 76).

Testing for Zinc Deficiency

You can do a simple zinc taste test to determine whether you have a zinc deficiency. This test is often available from health food shops and naturopathic clinics. Measure the recommended amount of liquid zinc and hold it in your mouth for a few seconds before swallowing it or spitting it out. Your taste buds will indicate the degree of need for zinc supplementation: if you have a deficiency, the mixture will taste like water, be pleasant tasting, or leave a furry feeling in the mouth. If your body has plenty of stored zinc, the liquid will taste metallic or foul and you'll probably want to spit it out.

Dosage Notes: Salt and supplements containing calcium, iron, and/or phosphorus can prevent zinc supplements from being absorbed, so, if possible, take your zinc supplement 1 to 2 hours apart from these substances.

Caution

Do not take zinc supplements if you have copper deficiency or if you are taking tetracycline (a drug for infections) because zinc competes for absorption with copper and may make your medical treatment less effective. Do not exceed the prescribed dosage because an excessive zinc intake can cause diarrhea, abdominal pains, nausea, dehydration, dizziness, and lethargy.

Powerful Co-Nutrients

The benefits of zinc can increase when taken with other nutrients.

- Zinc + magnesium + vitamin B6 + biotin (for delta-6-desaturase enzyme)
- Zinc + magnesium + B-group vitamins (to detoxify amines, hormones, and alcohol in Phase 2 liver detoxification)

Common Food Sources of Zinc

Food Source	Serving	Zinc Content
Oysters	12	54–76 mg approximately
Lamb shank, cooked	5 oz (150 g)	14.5 mg
Crab, cooked	3½ oz (100 g)	9.1 mg
Beef, cooked	5 oz (150 g)	7.7 mg
Lamb, cooked	5 oz (150 g)	6.4 mg
Dried beans	3½ oz (100 g)	3.0 mg
Brown rice	3½ oz (100 g)	2.1 mg
Muesli (granola)	2 oz (60 g)	1.8 mg
Shrimp, cooked	3½ oz (100 g)	1.8 mg
Peas	3½ oz (100 g)	1.8 mg
Wheat germ	2 tbsp (30 mL)	1.5 mg
Rolled (porridge) oats	2 oz (60 g)	1.1 mg
White rice	3½ oz (100 g)	1.1 mg
Whole wheat bread	2 slices	0.9 mg
White bread	2 slices	0.4 mg

Total Daily Intake of Zinc

Age Range	Total Daily Intake	Dosing
Adults	20 mg	Supplement form
5–17 years	10–15 mg	Supplement form
1–4 years	5 mg	Supplement form
0–12 months	2–4 mg	Obtain zinc through breast milk or infant formula

7. Chromium

The mineral chromium is required in micro amounts for normal growth and general health. In 1959, it was identified as the active ingredient in glucose tolerance factor. It enhances the action of the hormone insulin, which helps your body process glucose in the blood. Chromium is needed for the breakdown of proteins, carbohydrates, and fats, and it enhances the body's ability to convert glucose to energy. It is not a miracle nutrient or a "wonder" supplement, but for those who are deficient in chromium, supplementation can greatly improve energy levels, the ability to think clearly, and quality of life.

In the 1800s, carbohydrate avoidance was recommended as part of a diet that prevented eczema; however, with additional information about the benefits of chromium supplementation, total carbohydrate avoidance is not necessary or advised (because you need dietary fiber for gastrointestinal health). Chromium supplementation enables sufferers to be able to enjoy good-quality whole-grain carbohydrates while on the Eczema Diet.

Modern Western diets are low in chromium and generally rich in processed carbohydrates. Frequent sugar consumption is considered normal, causing an increased need for chromium in the diet. Chromium supplementation can decrease sugar cravings and cravings for carbohydrates and it can reduce excessive hunger, fatigue (especially after meals or during afternoon energy slumps), glucose intolerance, and irritability. Although statistics on chromium deficiency are limited, data from research suggest that only 0.4% to 2.5% of chromium is absorbed from foods. Vitamin C and vitamin B3 (niacin) enhance the absorption of chromium, as does protein, so take a chromium supplement with a protein-rich meal. Chromium picolinate is easier for the body to absorb than other types of chromium. A chromium supplement should also contain B6, B12, vitamin C, vitamin D3, folic acid, magnesium, and zinc.

Caution

If you are taking another prescription, consult with a nutritionist or doctor before taking chromium. If you have insulin-dependent diabetes, seek advice from your doctor before supplementing with chromium, because it alters blood sugar levels (insulin would need to be reduced if you were taking chromium, but do this only under your doctor's supervision).

Powerful Co-Nutrients

The benefits of chromium can increase when taken with other nutrients.

- Chromium + vitamin C + vitamin B3 + protein (to enhance absorption)

Common Food Sources of Chromium

Food Source	Serving	Chromium Content
Romaine lettuce	2 cups (500 mL)	15.6 mcg
Onion, raw	½ cup (125 mL)	12.4 mcg
Turkey	3½ oz (100 g)	10.4 mcg
Peas, cooked	1 cup (250 mL)	6.0 mcg
Dried garlic	1 tsp (5 mL)	3.0 mcg
Potato, mashed	1 cup (250 mL)	3.0 mcg
Whole wheat bread	2 slices	2.0 mcg
Banana	1 medium	1.0 mcg
Green beans	½ cup (125 mL)	1.0 mcg

Total Daily Intake of Chromium

Age Range	Total Daily Intake	Dosing
Adults	45 mcg	Supplement form
5–17 years	25 mcg	Supplement form
1–4 years	13 mcg	Supplement form
0–12 months	1–7 mcg	Obtain chromium through breast milk or infant formula

8. Vitamin D

Vitamin D is manufactured in two ways: in your skin after direct sunlight exposure and through your diet. It is an important fat-soluble vitamin that directly and indirectly controls more than 200 genes. According to research at the Boston Children's Hospital, children with moderate to severe atopic eczema have significantly lower levels of vitamin D compared with children who have mild symptoms. A study by the same researchers found that adults with eczema consume diets lower in vitamin D than people without eczema.

Vitamin D deficiency is common, especially in cooler climates. It is estimated that more than 1 billion people worldwide have vitamin D deficiency or insufficiency. Deficiency is linked to a

About 10 minutes every day of unfiltered sunshine directly on the skin will keep vitamin D deficiency away in healthy individuals.

range of health problems, including rickets, poor bone health, severe fatigue, psoriasis, muscle weakness, and a 30% to 50% increased risk of cancers of the colon, prostate, and breast.

What can diminish vitamin D in the body? Low or inadequate exposure to direct sunlight is the main contributing factor. This can occur in winter or cooler climates and from overuse of protective clothing and sunscreens. According to research published in the *British Journal of Dermatology*, frequent use of cortisone cream depletes vitamin D in the skin. When you use topical steroids or other topical drugs prescribed for eczema, you are advised to avoid direct sun exposure because topical steroids make the skin fragile and more prone to sun damage. This highlights another reason why we need to adopt healthy alternatives to medicated creams.

Enjoy safe sun exposure daily. About 10 minutes every day of unfiltered sunshine directly on the skin will keep vitamin D deficiency away in healthy individuals, but make sure adequate amounts of vitamin D are being consumed in your diet too. If you have eczema and/or vitamin D deficiency, a supplement is advised. Ask your doctor to check your vitamin D level.

Dosage Notes: Take vitamin D for 12 weeks, then halve the dosage or discontinue use. Vitamin D is measured in micrograms and international units: 1 mcg of vitamin D = 40 IU (international units). For example, 90 mcg = 3600 IU.

Caution

If you have diabetes, speak to your doctor before taking vitamin D because it may lower blood sugar levels. You may not be able to take vitamin D if you have kidney disease, kidney stones, or granulomatous disorders (immune disorder), because increased vitamin D intake may increase calcium in the blood.

Powerful Co-Nutrients

The benefits of vitamin D can increase when taken with other nutrients.

- Vitamin D + calcium + magnesium + vitamin K (for bone health)

Common Food Sources of Vitamin D

Food Source	Serving	Vitamin D Content
Herring, grilled	3½ oz (100 g)	25.0 mcg
Red salmon, canned	3½ oz (100 g)	23.1 mcg
Pink salmon, canned	3½ oz (100 g)	17.0 mcg
Trout, grilled	5 oz (150 g)	16.5 mcg
Salmon, grilled	5 oz (150 g)	14.4 mcg
Tuna, fresh	5 oz (150 g)	10.8 mcg
Kippers, cooked	3½ oz (100 g)	9.4 mcg
Mackerel, cooked	3½ oz (100 g)	5.4 mcg
Tuna, canned in brine	3½ oz (100 g)	3.0 mcg

Total Daily Intake of Vitamin D

Age Range	Total Daily Intake	Dosing
Adults	90 mcg (3600 IU)	Supplement form
5–17 years	30–60 mcg (1200–2400 IU)	Supplement form
1–4 years	15–30 mcg (600–1200 IU)	Supplement form
0–12 months	5–15 mcg (200–600 IU)	Obtain vitamin D through breast milk or infant formula

9. Vitamin E

Vitamin E is the predominant antioxidant in human skin. Supplementation can decrease the allergy marker immunoglobulin E (IgE) in allergy sufferers, improve immune responses, and decrease the production and release of pro-inflammatory prostaglandins. A clinical trial published in the *International Journal of Dermatology* revealed that nearly 50% of adults with atopic dermatitis who were treated with 400 IU (268 mg) of vitamin E daily for 8 months showed great improvement (compared to only one in the placebo group); and there was an almost complete remission of atopic eczema in seven people taking the vitamin E, but none in the placebo group (four of the adults treated with vitamin E worsened, compared to 36 in the placebo). Although this study showed promising results, other studies have not been so positive. It must be stressed that vitamin E should be taken with vitamin C and alpha-lipoic acid: you don't need to take the megadose of vitamin E used in this study (vitamin C and alpha-lipoic acid recycle vitamin E, helping it to circulate for longer).

Did You Know?

D-alpha-tocopherol

Vitamin E from natural food sources is called d-alpha-tocopherol. It is more potent than the synthetic form. Synthetic vitamin E is listed as dl-alpha-tocopherol, and this artificial form (denoted by "dl") should not be taken.

Dosage Notes: Take vitamin E (d-alpha-tocopherol) with vitamin C and alpha-lipoic acid.

Caution

Vitamin E thins the blood, so do not take vitamin E if you are on blood-thinning medications, such as aspirin, or if you are undergoing surgery. If you are on any medications, consult with your doctor before supplementing with vitamin E.

Powerful Co-Nutrients

The benefits of vitamin E can increase when taken with other nutrients.

- Vitamin E + vitamin C + alpha-lipoic acid (antioxidant protection)
- Vitamin E + quercetin (blocks pro-inflammatory leukotriene formation)

Common Food Sources of Vitamin E

1 IU (international unit) of vitamin E is equivalent to 0.67 mg of vitamin E. To convert IUs into mg (milligrams): multiply the number of IUs by 0.67.

Food Source	Serving	Vitamin E Content
Sunflower oil	4 tsp (20 mL)	9.8 mg
Cabbage	3½ oz (100 g)	0.2–7.0 mg*
Sweet potato	3½ oz (100 g)	4.6 mg
Salmon, grilled	5 oz (150 g)	3.5 mg
Shrimp	3½ oz (100 g)	2.9 mg
Soybeans, cooked	1 cup (250 mL)	2.2 mg
Chickpeas, cooked	1 cup (250 mL)	2.0 mg
Red salmon, canned	3½ oz (100 g)	2.1 mg
Tuna, canned in oil	3½ oz (100 g)	1.9 mg
Pink salmon, canned	3½ oz (100 g)	1.5 mg
Brussels sprouts	3½ oz (100 g)	1.0 mg
Leeks	3½ oz (100 g)	0.9 mg
Lettuce	3½ oz (100 g)	0.6 mg
Carrots, raw	½ cup	0.4 mg

*The green outer leaves of cabbage contain 7 mg of vitamin E; the white inner leaves have only 0.2 mg.

Total Daily Intake of Vitamin E

Age Range	Total Daily Intake	Dosing
Adults	80–100 mg (119–149 IU)	Supplement form
5–17 years	40–60 mg (60–90 IU)	Supplement form
1–4 years	20–30 mg (30–45 IU)	Supplement form
0–12 months	4–5 mg (6.0–7.5 IU)	Obtain vitamin E through breast milk or infant formula

10. Quercetin

Quercetin is a potent antioxidant flavonoid found in fruits and vegetables. It is the major therapeutic ingredient in onions and various herbal medicines. Quercetin is a natural antihistamine. It reduces blood histamine levels and it can help to reverse the liver damage caused by nitrate consumption. When combined with vitamin C, it can quickly reduce and prevent hay fever symptoms. Quercetin is anti-inflammatory, meaning that it inhibits formation of pro-inflammatory leukotrienes, which are associated with eczema and asthma (see "How Prostaglandins Control Inflammation," page 46).

Dosage Notes: Do not take quercetin as a single supplement. Instead, take it in a multivitamin formula that includes vitamin C, and take it in divided doses with food. For example, adults can have 40 mg of quercetin twice daily, with breakfast and lunch.

Safety

Quercetin supplementation is generally safe. High doses of quercetin (of 150 mg or more) can cause side effects, including low blood pressure, headaches, upset stomach, numbness, and tingling, and may interfere with some medical drugs. If you have kidney disease, avoid quercetin and other supplements.

Do not take quercetin if you are taking corticosteroids or cyclosporine. Avoid high-dose quercetin if you are taking blood-thinning medications, such as aspirin or warfarin. If you are undergoing chemotherapy, talk to your doctor before taking quercetin.

Common Food Sources of Quercetin

Food Source	Serving	Quercetin Content
Buckwheat	3½ oz (100 g)	15.0–36.0 mg
Elderberries, raw	1½ oz (50 g)	21.0 mg
Onions, cooked	1½ oz (50 g)	9.9 mg
Buckwheat groats, roasted	3½ oz (100 g)	2.0–8.7 mg
Blueberries, raw or frozen	3½ oz (100 g)	2.0–7.3 mg
Green onions, raw	1½ oz (50 g)	7.1 mg
Apple, with skin	3½ oz (100 g)	4.4 mg
Celery, raw	3½ oz (100 g)	3.5 mg
Yellow beans, snap, raw	3½ oz (100 g)	3.0 mg
Buckwheat flour	3½ oz (100 g)	2.7 mg
Green beans, raw	3½ oz (100 g)	2.7 mg
Lettuce, iceberg	3½ oz (100 g)	2.4 mg
Cherries, canned	1½ oz (50 g)	1.6 mg
Apple, peeled	3½ oz (100 g)	1.5 mg
Bilberries, raw	1½ oz (50 g)	1.5 mg
Green beans, frozen, cooked	3½ oz (100 g)	1.2 mg
Pear, raw	3½ oz (100 g)	0.4 mg

Total Daily Intake of Quercetin

Age Range	Total Daily Intake	Dosing
Adults	80–130 mg	Supplement form
5–17 years	40–60 mg	Supplement form
1–4 years	10 mg	Supplement form
0–12 months		Obtain quercetin through breast milk or infant formula, or by consuming solids

11. Alpha-Lipoic Acid

Alpha-lipoic acid, also known as lipoic acid and thioctic acid, is made in small quantities by a healthy body and it has the unique talent of being both water- and fat-soluble. In animal studies, alpha-lipoic acid supplementation increases the formation of the powerful antioxidant glutathione, which is essential for healthy skin and the liver's detoxification of chemicals, toxic metals, antibiotics, and alcohol. Alpha-lipoic acid regenerates other antioxidants, including vitamin C and vitamin E, and it assists with converting glucose (blood sugar) into energy.

Common Food Sources of Alpha-Lipoic Acid
- Brussels sprouts
- Potatoes
- Rice bran

Sources not suitable while you have eczema
- Spinach
- Broccoli
- Peas
- Brewer's yeast
- Asparagus
- Organ meats

Total Daily Intake of Alpha-Lipoic Acid

Age Range	Total Daily Intake	Dosing
Adults	45–50 mg	Supplement form
5–17 years	15–25 mg	Supplement form
1–4 years	5–10 mg	Supplement form
0–12 months		Obtain alpha-lipoic acid through breast milk or infant formula

Dosage Notes: Take alpha-lipoic acid with vitamins C and E as a part of a multivitamin formula.

Caution

If you have diabetes or hypoglycemia, be cautious when taking alpha-lipoic acid, because it lowers blood sugar and may cause hypoglycemia. If you are taking drugs to lower blood sugar, such as insulin, do not take alpha-lipoic acid without consulting your physician.

12. Essential Fatty Acids

Essential fatty acids (EFAs) are vital for healthy skin and are classified as essential fats because your body cannot manufacture them and they must be obtained from your diet. The two main groups of essential fatty acids are omega-3 and omega-6. Rich sources of omega-3 include flax seeds and fish, especially trout, salmon, and sardines. (See "Safe Seafood," page 69.)

Omega-3 Dosage Guidelines

Eczema sufferers may not digest or utilize fats adequately due to genetics or faulty enzyme conversions.

- Eczema sufferers should obtain their omega-3 from food sources rather than taking a supplement because omega-3 is better absorbed from foods.
- If you experience beneficial effects from taking fish oil supplements, look for supplements that are unflavored and color-free (children's fish oil supplements usually contain natural or artificial flavors, so they are not eczema-safe).
- Eat eczema-safe fish twice a week (see "Safe Seafood," page 69).
- Consume whole or ground flax seeds or fresh flaxseed oil daily. Flaxseed oil and oil supplements should be taken with soy lecithin granules to increase absorption (lecithin information is on page 71). Recipes include Healthy Skin Smoothie (page 209) in Stage 1, and in Stage 2 only, Flaxseed Lemon Drink (page 208).
- EPA (eicosapentaenoic acid) and DHA (docosahexaenoic acid) are omega-3 EFAs in their converted and more potent form. Many of the health benefits of omega-3 are attributed to EPA and DHA.
- EPA and DHA are also present in the foods listed on page 118, especially cold-water fish.

Dosage Notes: In fish, the EPA and DHA content varies depending on whether the skin has been left on or removed: fish with skin on are higher in fat, so they are richer sources of omega-3 fatty acids EPA and DHA.

Skin Moisture

To demonstrate how diet influences the skin, a group of research scientists gave one group of women flaxseed oil, another group borage oil, and a third group a placebo, which was olive oil, for 12 weeks. After 6 weeks of consuming ½ teaspoon (2 mL) of either flaxseed oil or borage oil, skin water loss was decreased by about 10%, and by week 12, the flaxseed-oil group showed further protection from water loss and the skin was significantly more hydrated. Although the olive oil (placebo) group had no significant change, at 12 weeks, the flaxseed oil group had significantly less skin reddening (after irritation), roughness, and scaling of the skin.

Other EFAs do not have this moisturizing effect. Olive oil contains mostly omega-9 EFAs, which do not influence skin hydration, and saturated fats from meat and dairy products actually promote dry skin in eczema sufferers. Research shows that diets high in fats, where 10% of energy is consumed as saturated fat and monounsaturated fat (from vegetable oils, margarine, and nuts), decrease skin hydration and increase the skin's surface pH, making the skin more susceptible to microbe invasion and bacterial infections.

Common Food Sources of Omega-3 Essential Fatty Acids

Food Source	Serving	Omega-3 Content
Salmon	4 oz (113 g)	2000 mg
Flax seeds	1 tbsp (15 mL)	1750 mg
Omega-3 fortified eggs	2	1114 mg
Scallops	4 oz (113 g)	1100 mg
Soybeans	1 cup (250 mL)	700 mg
Halibut, baked	4 oz (113 g)	620 mg
Tofu	4 oz (113 g)	360 mg
Baby (pattypan) squash	1 cup (250 mL)	340 mg
Cabbage	1 cup (250 mL)	170 mg

Common Food Sources of EPA and DHA

Food Source	Serving	EPA / DHA Content
Atlantic salmon	3½ oz (100 g)	1090–1830 mg*
Tuna, fresh	3½ oz (100 g)	240–1280 mg*
Herring	3½ oz (100 g)	1710–1810 mg*
Sardines	3½ oz (100 g)	980–1700 mg*
Mackerel	3½ oz (100 g)	340–1570 mg*
Rainbow trout	3½ oz (100 g)	840–980 mg
Flaxseed oil	1 tbsp (15 mL)	850 mg
Tuna, canned in water, drained	3½ oz (100 g)	260–730 mg*
Flax seeds, ground or whole	1 tbsp (15 mL)	220 mg
Soy flaxseed bread	2 slices	180 mg

*The EPA and DHA content varies depending on whether the skin has been left on or removed; fish with skin on are higher in fat, so they are richer sources of EPA and DHA.

13. Probiotics

Probiotics contain health-promoting bacteria, also known as microflora, which are naturally found in the gastrointestinal tract of healthy people. At birth, an infant's gastrointestinal tract contains no bacteria — it is sterile — then, during the first year of life, colonization begins and (ideally) a healthy range of bacteria is established. Microflora work by adhering to your gut wall and "policing" potentially harmful microbes so they can't multiply and thrive. Beneficial bacteria promote healthy digestion and they can manufacture some vitamins, including the B-group vitamins, so they help to decrease the risk of nutritional deficiencies.

Unfortunately, beneficial microflora are not always present in adequate amounts. Microflora imbalance or deficiency is associated with antibiotic use, illness, diarrhea, and poor health of the gastrointestinal tract. Microflora imbalance allows pathogens, such as *Candida albicans*, to thrive in the gastrointestinal tract and this increases the risk of food intolerances and itchy skin. Research shows that an altered ratio of the microflora strains can precede the development of atopic eczema. According to one study, the presence of the bacterial strains *Escherichia coli* and *Clostridium difficile* is associated with an increased risk of eczema and allergies at 2 years of age. The research suggests that probiotics can promote proper gut barrier function and the healing of intestinal permeability. In some (but not all) studies, probiotics decreased allergic inflammation in eczema sufferers.

Microflora Imbalances

The signs that indicate you may have a microflora imbalance or deficiency include:

- Skin inflammation
- Itchy skin
- *Candida albicans* infestation (symptoms are listed in the *Candida albicans* questionnaire, page 42)
- Allergies and increased sensitivities
- Cravings for sugar
- White fungal patches on the skin
- Biotin deficiency (and other B-group vitamins)
- Gastrointestinal dysfunction (diarrhea or constipation, foul-smelling gas and/or stools, bloating, abdominal pain, poor digestion)

Associated Conditions

These symptoms can also be caused by other conditions and should be discussed with your doctor. Microflora imbalance can be caused by or is associated with the following factors:

- Cesarean or premature birth
- Candida infection in the vaginal tract at the time of birth
- Use of oral antibiotics
- Diarrhea
- Compromised gut function
- Gut lining permeability
- High-sugar diets (acid-promoting diets)
- Immune system dysfunction
- Use of the birth control pill
- Hormone replacement therapy
- Corticosteroids (e.g., hydrocortisone)
- Excessive consumption of processed foods, including refined carbohydrates (white bread, cake, cookies, sodas), sugar (including in sodas, cordial, fruit juice)
- Frequent consumption of alcohol

Types of Microflora

The beneficial bacteria in probiotics come from two groups of microflora: lactobacillus and bifidobacterium. Within these groups are different strains, such as *Lactobacillus acidophilus* and *Bifidobacterium animalis*. The benefits from probiotics are strain-specific. For example, the strain *L. acidophilus* LA-5 does not treat eczema (it helps conditions such as *Candida albicans*), but the strain known as *L. rhamnosus* GG was found to improve eczema symptoms in children with eczema.

Probiotics should be used after an eczema sufferer has taken a course of antibiotics, been ill, had diarrhea, experienced an adverse or allergic reaction to food, or if the sufferer has compromised gut function, dandruff, *Candida albicans*, or fungal infestation. When choosing a probiotic supplement, look at the ingredients panel for the specific strain of probiotic (for example, *L. rhamnosus* GG). Probiotics are generally safe for infants, but speak to your physician or dietitian about dosage and safety.

Probiotics for Eczema and Associated Conditions

Condition	Suitable Probiotic Strain
Eczema	*Lactobacillus rhamnosus* GG (also known as LGG or *Lactobacillus* GG) *Bifidobacterium animalis*, (also known as *B. lactis* Bb12 or *Bifidobacterium lactis* Bb12) *Lactobacillus fermentum* PCC *Lactobacillus reuteri* ATCC 55730 *Lactobacillus reuteri* DSM 122460 (combined with *Lactobacillus rhamnosus* GG)
Candida albicans	*Lactobacillus acidophilus* LA-5 *Lactobacillus rhamnosus* GG *Lactobacillus acidophilus*, strain NAS *Lactobacillus acidophilus* NCFM
Digestive dysfunction	*Lactobacillus rhamnosus* GG *Bifidobacterium lactis* Bb12 (also known as *Bifidobacterium animalis* Bb12) *Lactobacillus johnsonii* La1 *Lactobacillus plantarum* 299v *Lactobacillus paracasei* Shirota *Propionibacterium freudenreichii* HA-101 and HA-102 Sauerkraut (probiotic food)
Antibiotics	*Lactobacillus rhamnosus* GG *Lactobacillus acidophilus* LA-5
Allergies	*Lactobacillus rhamnosus* GG *Lactobacillus johnsonii* La1

Dosage notes: Take a suitable probiotic supplement twice daily, mixed in a little water or rice milk, before breakfast and in the afternoon. If serving probiotics to small children, you can also sprinkle probiotic grains onto cold cereal or cooled baby rice cereal (don't add probiotics to overly warm foods), or add it to their milk bottle after the milk has been warmed.

Caution

Discontinue use of probiotics if diarrhea or constipation occurs.

14. Carotenoids

Research shows that eating foods rich in cryptoxanthin, a carotenoid that supplies vitamin A, can help to increase skin hydration when consumed as a part of a healthy diet. Fat-soluble vitamin A has the opposite effect — it dries out the skin — and should not be taken in supplement form unless vitamin A deficiency has been diagnosed. Cryptoxanthin-rich foods include papaya, which can be consumed daily. It is also rich in vitamin C. Other carotenoid-rich foods that are eczema-safe and vital for eczema sufferers include carrots, beets, and sweet potato. Have at least one carotenoid-rich fruit or vegetable daily.

15. Calcium

Calcium is the most abundant mineral in the body. It is stored in your bones. The body regulates a constant level of calcium in the blood in order to keep the blood pH slightly alkaline, and this is beneficial for bone and skin health. In one study, calcium helped to improve the acid mantle of the skin. However, high calcium intake can interfere with iron and zinc absorption. Paradoxically, dairy products contribute to eczema, while calcium in supplement form is beneficial, boosting moisture levels in the skin. Indeed, it is essential to take a calcium supplement while on the Eczema Diet. Calcium is best taken when combined with vitamin D, and taken separately from iron.

A calcium supplement can be taken just before breakfast and lunch or as prescribed by your doctor.

Common Food Sources of Calcium

Food Source	Serving	Calcium Content
Calcium-fortified soy milk or rice milk	1 cup (250 mL)	300 mg
Sardines, canned or fresh	3½ oz (100 g)	300 mg
Salmon, canned or fresh	3½ oz (100 g)	200–300 mg
Soybeans, cooked	½ cup (125 mL)	130 mg
Oatmeal/porridge	1 bowl	99–110 mg
Fish fillet	5½ oz (160 g)	85 mg
Rainbow trout, cooked	2½ oz (75 g)	73 mg
Cabbage	3½ oz (100 g)	40 mg

Recommended Calcium Intake from Supplements and Food

Age Range	Daily Calcium Intake
Adults	1000 mg
During pregnancy, lactation or menopause	1200 mg
5–17 years old	800 mg
1–4 years old	500 mg
Infants 7–12 months old	270 mg

Caution

Combined dietary and supplemental intake of calcium should not exceed 2500 mg daily because excessive calcium can cause adverse reactions. Do not take calcium if you have kidney failure, kidney stones, hyperparathyroidism, sarcoidosis, or cancer. Calcium supplementation can interfere with medications, so speak to your doctor if you take medications. Do not take antacids containing aluminum, because calcium can significantly increase the amount of aluminum absorbed into the blood. If you need antacids, this may be a sign your diet is too high in acidifying foods (see "Restore Your Acid-Alkaline Balance," page 55).

> Keep in mind that you need vitamin A in your diet to avoid deficiency and you will obtain a safe amount of vitamin A from red meat, chicken, seafood, and orange-colored vegetables.

Supplements to Avoid or Limit

The following is a list of the supplements best avoided by those with eczema.

Herbal Supplements

All herbal medicines, including milk thistle (which is in most liver detoxification supplements), are rich in natural plant chemicals, such as salicylates. Green tea (in both tea form and in supplements), vegetable extracts, broccoli, wheat grass juice, and barley grass all contain very high levels of salicylates. They are not eczema-safe.

Vitamin A

Fat-soluble vitamin A (retinol) helps to mop up excess oil in the skin, so it decreases skin moisture, which is beneficial if you have acne but not good for eczema and dry skin. High intake of vitamin A is associated with a significant increase in surface pH (in women), and this is not good for eczema sufferers, who need a lower, acidic pH to guard against invading bacteria. For this reason, eczema sufferers should not take a supplement containing vitamin A or cod liver oil, or eat liver, without first consulting a dietitian.

Keep in mind that you need vitamin A in your diet to avoid deficiency and you will obtain a safe amount of vitamin A from red meat, chicken, seafood, and orange-colored vegetables.

Guidelines for Taking Supplements

This is a wide range of supplements and not all of them are absolutely essential to take during the program and all at one time (for example, fish oil supplements). So to avoid confusion, here are the main supplements recommended in the Eczema Diet. Use this list to buy your supplements at your pharmacy and check off each nutrient you take on a daily basis. Once your eczema improves, you should be able to reduce the dosages, but check with your physician or dietitian before changing dosage. If you need extra assistance finding supplements for eczema, go to my website at www.healthbeforebeauty.com.

- Vitamin C
- Glycine
- Vitamin B6
- Magnesium
- Vitamin E
- Biotin
- Zinc
- Calcium
- Alpha-lipoic acid
- Quercetin
- Vitamin D3
- Chromium
- Omega-3 essential fatty acids
- Probiotics
- Vitamin K is also recommended to balance this formula

Part 4

Healthy Skin Care Routine

Chapter 6
Skin Care Products

Testimonial

My 16-month-old son Jagger has suffered with eczema since birth, especially on his feet and behind his knees. After I put him on Karen's anti-eczema program, within a couple of days, he was sleeping better and scratching less. Within 10 days, all the redness was gone from his skin and I could leave him without clothes, and without scratching! He's much happier and busy playing instead of scratching!

Karma Montagne

Did You Know?

First Recorded Treatment

"On the first day, the head was painted with a lotion of durrameal and fruit-of-the-dompalm, warmed in soft fat, and was bound up. On the second day, the head was anointed with fish oil; on the fourth day, with abra oil. After this course of intensive treatment, the offending head, if the eczema still persisted, was smeared daily with breadmeal and dressed with rotted cereals." This is the first recorded treatment for eczema, found in a papyrus dating from ancient Egypt.

When you start the Eczema Diet Program, you may not see results instantly. It may take a few weeks before you notice your skin healing. Until then, and perhaps for some time afterward, you may want to use skin care products, including moisturizers and body washes. Your skin is constructed, repaired, and maintained using nutrients obtained from your daily diet. However, when you have eczema, a little extra help from the outside is a welcome relief. A healthy skin care routine can speed up the healing process and soothe the itch, but if you are not careful, the wrong skin care routine can damage the barrier function of the skin and delay healing.

Problematic Skin Care Ingredients

There is not one definitive group of skin care ingredients that will be eczema-safe for everyone. One eczema patient will say that plain sorbolene cream is the only product her skin can tolerate, while another will find sorbolene cream irritates her skin and she

Problematic Skin Care Products

Skin Care Product	Uses/Found In	Problems
Sulfates		
Sodium lauryl sulfate (SLS) is especially problematic; milder sulfates include sodium laureth sulfate, sodium C14-16 olefin sulfonate, TEA-lauryl sulfate	Found in foaming detergents, emulsifiers, toiletries, aqueous creams, commercial toothpastes, shampoos, cleansers, hand wash, baby shampoos, and bubble bath	SLS causes contact dermatitis, alters the skin's pH, thins the skin barrier (damage can last for 4 weeks), and causes water loss from the skin, rashes, dandruff, hair loss, and dry skin
Formaldehyde		
Formaldehyde and its derivatives imidazolidinyl urea and DMDM hydantoin	Used as a preservative; found in shampoos, liquid hand soap, hair products, hair gels, cosmetics, nail polish, and moisturizers	Releases formaldehyde and causes skin irritation, allergic reactions, and rashes; it may affect breathing in asthmatics
Fragrance		
More than 4,000 varieties of synthetic fragrances and eaux de parfum	Used to hide undesirable smells; found in moisturizers, cosmetics, deodorant, cleansers, hair conditioners, shampoos, baby shampoo, perfumes, cosmetics, and colognes	Aggravates hand eczema and dermatitis; can cause dizziness, hyper-pigmentation of the skin, hyperactivity, and irritation in children and some adults
Isopropyl alcohol (isopropanol)		
	Used as an antibacterial solvent made from petroleum toners; found in shaving creams and other men's skin care products	It is drying and irritating; strips the skin's natural acid mantle, making it vulnerable to bacteria and fungus; promotes liver spots and pigmentation; and can irritate the eyes and skin
Diethanolamine (DEA) and monoethanolamide (MEA)		
Such as lauramide DEA, cocamide DEA, and cocamide MEA	Used as an emulsifier to mix oil and water and as a foaming agent in shampoos	Can cause contact allergies, such as skin rashes

instead uses natural, herbal-based moisturizers for relief. When you have eczema, it is essential to keep your skin care regimen simple and avoid using topical products that can irritate the skin. Always read the label carefully and check the ingredients before buying products for your skin. While you have eczema, there are many ways to minimize your discomfort. Some of the following information is age-specific and specific to certain living arrangements, so take from this list what is relevant to you.

Beneficial Skin Care Ingredients

The following ingredients work best when used within a skin care product that contains a range of ingredients, but it is not necessary or advised to use all these ingredients at once. If your skin is broken, irritation can occur, so always test a product on undamaged skin before applying it to your eczema.

Creams and Lotions

These products are thin in consistency and rapidly soak into the skin. However, creams and lotions need to be reapplied more often and they may not offer enough protection for very dry and itchy skin.

Essential Oils

Natural essential oils blended into an eczema cream may be beneficial for the skin, but keep in mind they can also cause skin irritation, especially if you are sensitive to salicylates.

Emollients

Various types of moisturizers are collectively referred to as emollients. The following emollients, presented from thickest to thinnest in consistency, can help to make shopping for a skin care product easier. Before purchasing an emollient, check the ingredient list and, if possible, test it on a patch of healthy, unbroken skin to see if irritation occurs.

Ointments

Ointments, such as petroleum and papaya ointment, are thick and greasy, making them useful for scaly skin and extremely dry patches. A thick coat of ointment can protect your skin from stinging when you go for a swim in the ocean or a chlorinated

> **Did You Know?**
> ....
> **Contamination**
> Unpreserved or poorly preserved skin care products can become contaminated with bacteria and can lead to bacterial infections if you have broken skin. To reduce the risk of contaminating your skin care products, do not put your fingers into pots of ointment or skin creams, and throw out older products. Although there is a risk of stinging from preserved skin care products, favor products that are preserved.

Beneficial Skin Care Products

Ingredient	Properties
Aloe vera	Anti-inflammatory, antibacterial
Black currant seed oil (*Ribes nigrum*)	Anti-inflammatory; has moisturizing properties; contains omega-3
Borage oil	Anti-inflammatory; contains gamma-linolenic acid (GLA) and omega-3
Calendula (*Calendula officinalis*)	Anti-inflammatory, antiseptic, antibacterial, and astringent; contains flavonoids
Chamomile (*Anthemis nobilis*)	Astringent, antibacterial, anti-inflammatory; contains fatty acids, rutin, and quercetin
Cocoa butter	Has moisturizing properties; contains antioxidants, such as vitamin E
Emu oil	Anti-inflammatory; contains omega-3 fatty acids
Evening primrose oil	Anti-inflammatory; contains gamma-linolenic acid (GLA)
Jojoba oil	Protects skin from water loss; similar to your skin's own sebum
Licorice root/licorice extract (*Glycyrrhiza glabra*)	Anti-inflammatory, antiviral, antibacterial
Manuka honey	Anti-inflammatory, antibacterial, and moisturizing; contains antioxidants
Rose hip oil (good-quality rose hip oil should be a rich amber color)	Moisturizing; contains antioxidants, vitamin C, all trans-retinoic acid (natural vitamin A), lycopene, carotenoids, and essential fatty acids
Sea buckthorn berry oil	Anti-inflammatory, moisturizing; contains antioxidants (vitamin A, C, and E) and palmitoleic acid (a fatty acid in human skin sebum); has a unique 1:1 ratio of omega-3 and omega-6 oils
Shea butter (*Butyrospermum parkii*)	Very moisturizing; contains fatty acids and a small amount of natural UV factor; anti-inflammatory
Vitamin E, natural (d-alpha-tocopherol or tocopherol)	Is a natural preservative and antioxidant (do not use oils that are 100% vitamin E oil because they may cause pigmentation of the skin, and avoid synthetic "dl" vitamin E, such as dl-alpha-tocopherol)

pool (it is best to avoid chlorine if you can help it). Be cautious, though. Ointments can stain your clothes and they can cause rebound dryness when you stop using the product. Vaseline and papaya ointments are petroleum-based, but there are petroleum-free papaya ointments available.

According to the National Eczema Society in the United Kingdom, ointments do not contain preservatives, so they should not be used on weeping eczema or broken skin. Avoid putting your fingers into the pot of ointment because bacterial contamination can occur. Use a clean utensil to transfer some of the ointment into another clean container before applying.

Moisturizers

Studies show that damaged skin barrier function can be partially restored by applying oil-based moisturizers because they contain fatty acids and other nutrients and help to prevent water loss. However, moisturizers may not be protective enough for very dry and irritated skin. When eczema flares up, a non-irritating moisturizer can be applied two to four times daily, and in severe cases up to six times daily.

Washes and Soaps

Normal, healthy skin should have a pH of 5.5, but after soap use, the pH increases to more than 7.5. This is because most soaps and cleansing products are highly alkaline (with a pH range of 9 to 11). Most cleansing products also contain sulfates, which disrupt the skin's protective acid mantle and break down the skin's valuable barrier. Skin cleansers, soaps, detergents, and other foaming agents can cause dryness, swelling, flaking, tightness, roughness, and thinning of the skin barrier and they can leave the skin vulnerable to microbes, irritants, and allergens.

Body Washes

Body washes usually come in liquid soap form, which foams when friction is applied. Babies with eczema do not generally need to be washed with a body wash because it may irritate their eczema. If necessary, use sensitive-skin body washes to cleanse under the arms and feet, and to wash dirty hands. Look for products that are labeled "sulfate-free" and contain no sodium lauryl sulfate; they should also have a balanced pH of 5 to 6. These products should be low-foaming or non-foaming.

Facial Cleansers

Cleansers are used to dislodge dirt, pollution, and makeup. The risk with using a foaming cleanser is that it may contain ingredients that strip the skin's natural oils, giving your skin a "squeaky clean" effect. If your skin feels tight and dry after cleansing, then the product is too harsh. A good cleanser can remove dirt and pollution without stripping your skin of all of its protective sebum.

Look for non-foaming cleansers labeled "sulfate-free" that feel creamy, not soapy, and that are non-bubbly when applied to the skin. Pure almond oil or jojoba oil can be used to remove makeup and, like all products, you should discontinue use if an adverse reaction occurs.

Toners

A well-designed toner can help to restore the natural acidic pH of the skin. However, toners can cause skin irritations, so do not apply them to eczema or sensitive skin. Skip the toner in your beauty routine and spend your money on a good moisturizer instead.

Makeup Guidelines

Makeup can have a place in your skin care routine if you choose.

1. **Use fresh products.** Be aware that all products deteriorate over time, and bacteria from your fingers can contaminate makeup products, which might infect your eczema. As a general rule, makeup should be replaced within 3 years after leaving the factory. Natural makeup products that use natural preservatives, such as herbs, will have a shorter use-by date, so if using these products, refer to the packaging for further details (there will probably be a symbol of a container with an opened lid and below it a reference to how many months it will last once opened). When a product deteriorates, you might see mold or a change in texture, consistency, and/or smell.

2. **Avoid natural products that don't use preservatives.** There is an increased risk of bacterial contamination when you have eczema or broken skin.

3. **Clean your brushes and applicators.** When you have broken skin, hygiene is very important, so wash your makeup brushes and other applicators once a week to remove bacteria.

Preserving Skin Care Products

Skin Care Product	Lifespan	Tip
Blush and eye shadow	1–2 years	Wash brushes regularly using hand soap and warm water
Cleanser	6–12 months (refer to packaging)	Use non-foaming cleansers containing anti-inflammatory oils
Facial powder, eyeliner, and lipstick	2 years	Don't share makeup
Foundation and concealer	12–18 months	Fingers can hasten bacterial contamination
Mascara	3–6 months	This has a short lifespan because the pumping action can push bacteria to the bottom of the container
Moisturizer	3–12 months (refer to packaging)	Fingers dipped into a moisturizer tub can hasten bacterial contamination; enclosed pump or pourable containers are best

Deodorants and Antiperspirants

Sprayed or rolled on deodorants use fragrance, alcohol, and chemicals to mask body odor. Antiperspirants can contain chemicals, parabens, and aluminum, and work by affecting the sweat gland to prevent sweating.

Avoid chemical antiperspirants and use sensitive-skin deodorants when necessary: for example, if exercising or in hot weather. Most days, opt for a natural mineral salt deodorant (they look like a shaped crystal or a smooth salt rock). When moistened and rubbed under your arms, the minerals stop odor-causing bacteria. They are aluminum-free, hypoallergenic, fragrance-free, and paraben-free. If you have eczema in your armpits, avoid all forms of deodorants and instead use a moisturizer and dietary changes to improve your symptoms.

Sunscreen

Protect eczema from excess sun exposure because sunburn can cause skin damage. However, in sensitive individuals, sunscreens can cause irritation if applied directly onto eczema. If using sunscreen, favor sensitive-skin sunscreens formulated for children and babies (because they are generally lower in chemicals than regular sunscreens) and avoid sunscreens that are artificially colored.

Protect your skin with clothing and a hat and apply sunscreen on unaffected areas, but remember that some sun exposure, free of sunscreen, is necessary for healthy skin, and 10 minutes of direct sunlight on the skin daily is enough to prevent vitamin D deficiency.

Q. I've tried eczema creams before and they always sting my skin. How do I know if a skin product is right for me?

A. Test all skin care products on undamaged skin first. When testing an emollient on undamaged skin, if your skin swells or burns, or feels hot, tingly, or slightly more irritated, then the moisturizer is not right for you. If your skin peels or flakes, then the product is not suitable for you either. If a reaction occurs, wash the product off and apply something soothing, such as plain ointment.

If no reaction occurs after testing a product on undamaged skin, then apply a small amount of moisturizer to one patch of your eczema. Because your skin is damaged, this is likely to sting. Stinging may last between 1 and 3 minutes and you should stop reacting to a cream within three applications. For example, if you apply the moisturizer twice daily, then by the end of the second day, your skin should not sting at all. If your skin continues to hurt after the fourth application, then you are probably reacting to an ingredient and you should wash the emollient off and discontinue use.

Daily Skin Care Regimen

Here is an example of a simple face-cleansing regimen for morning and evening.

Morning

1. Wash hands with a gentle hand wash to remove bacteria, then rinse with water.

2. Have a brief warm shower or bath for 5 to 10 minutes. Add oil to bath if desired (see "Bath Recipes," page 136). Alternatively, fill a basin or large bowl with warm water and splash your face and neck four to six times.

3. After wetting your skin, gently pat with a soft cotton towel until your skin is nearly, but not quite, dry.

4. Immediately apply a suitable emollient or moisturizer to your skin.

Evening

1. Wash your hands with a gentle hand wash to remove bacteria, then rinse with water.

2. Have a brief warm shower or bath for 5 to 10 minutes. Add oil to bath if desired (see "Bath Recipes," page 136). Alternatively, fill a basin or large bowl with warm water and splash your face and neck four to six times.

3. If you are removing makeup, have been exercising, or have soiled skin, use a non-foaming cleanser and gently pat it onto your face and neck (babies and children do not need a cleanser, but they might occasionally need a gentle children's wash that is free of harsh ingredients (see "Body Washes," page 131).

4. Then, if cleansing, wet a cotton pad or ball, or use a very soft facial cloth, and gently wipe off the cleanser, pollution, and makeup (if relevant).

5. Thoroughly rinse off the cleanser with warm water.

6. Gently pat your skin with a soft cotton towel until your skin is almost dry. Immediately apply a suitable emollient.

Did You Know?

Over-Cleaning

If you cleansed your face the night before, you don't need to use a cleanser in the morning; it's better to avoid over-cleaning your face so that your natural oils can work their magic.

Bath Recipes

Bathing can be a useful way to temporarily relieve dry, itchy skin, and adding oil to the water coats the skin and can help to lock in moisture. Depending on the severity of your eczema, use warm bath water (not hot) and soak for less than 10 minutes so you don't dry out your skin. After bathing, pat your skin semi-dry with a soft towel and then apply a suitable moisturizer. When choosing a bath oil, look for eczema-safe ingredients, such as evening primrose oil, emu oil, jojoba oil, and borage oil. Avoid any bath products that bubble or contain sulfates.

Effective and Safe Bath Recipes

These recipes can be used in a standard-sized bath, filled one-third with water. Adjust the measurements according to the depth and size of your bath.

Bicarb Bath Recipe

This recipe is especially useful for babies and it can temporarily relieve the itch.

1. Add $\frac{1}{4}$ cup (60 mL) baking soda to warm bath water.
2. Bathe for 5 to 10 minutes.

Moisturizing Bath Recipe

Evening primrose oil is used as an example in this recipe; however, you can test a range of oils to see which one is best for your skin.

1. Mix together 1 teaspoon (5 mL) evening primrose oil or oil of choice (for a child's bath, use 1 capsule, pierced) and 1 tablespoon (15 mL) of your favorite emollient/moisturizer. The moisturizer helps the oil to diffuse more easily.
2. Disperse the mixture into a warm bath.
3. Bathe for 5 to 10 minutes.

Salt Bath Recipe

Bathing in the ocean can help promote healing of the skin, so if you live near the sea (and can brave the sting), have a swim. Alternatively, have a salt bath using Epsom salts, which are rich in magnesium. This salt bath is mild but it still may sting. This recipe is suitable for adults.

1. Add $\frac{1}{4}$ cup (60 mL) Epsom salts and $\frac{1}{4}$ cup (60 mL) sea salt (use less if desired) to a warm bath and briefly dissolve the crystals.
2. Soak for 10 minutes.
3. Rinse off the salt with water before patting skin semi-dry and moisturizing immediately.

Creating an Eczema-Safe Home

The environment you live in can irritate sensitive skin, but changes can be made to create an eczema-safe home.

Eight Tips for a Healthy Home Environment

Mold

Clean up the growth of any mold in damp areas and prevent further growth by placing moisture absorbers or dehumidifiers, available from most hardware stores, in all damp areas.

Cigarette Smoke

Forbid cigarette smoking indoors.

Heating and Cooling

Use electric heating and air-conditioning sparingly because they dry out the skin. If this is not possible, frequently apply an emollient to your skin to minimize moisture loss.

Chemical Exposure

- Avoid pesticide and chemical exposures on farms that use crop spraying.
- Steer clear of busy, polluted roads.
- Do not use unnatural chemical cleaning products and do not use nail polish.

- Avoid formaldehyde in new carpets, new cars, and new office and home furniture.
- If you are exposed to chemicals, eat a variety of alkalizing eczema-healthy vegetables and take antioxidants to help the liver detoxify these chemicals.
- Ventilate the house by opening the windows each day, to help disperse chemicals released from furnishings.

Recipes for Natural Cleaning Products

Vinegar Cleaning Spray

Vinegar is naturally antibacterial and it cuts through grease, making it a good all-purpose cleaning spray for kitchen countertops, toilets, baths, and tabletops. Do not use vinegar on marble surfaces. Cheap plastic spray bottles, bought from the discount shop, may buckle out of shape when vinegar is placed in it for prolonged periods. Instead, recycle an old cleaning product spray bottle; these are generally made with stronger plastic.

1. Empty spray bottle.
2. Add equal parts water and white vinegar to the bottle.
3. Mix the contents.

Baking Soda Scrub

Baking soda, from the baking section in most supermarkets, makes a handy (and cheap) all-purpose scrub. Sprinkle some onto a damp cloth and use it to clean bathroom and kitchen surfaces. Along with a scrubbing brush, it's perfect for cleaning the bath.

Bedding

You are likely sensitive to some fabrics that you find to be itchy, and while you have broken skin, you may be sensitive to dust mites. Try these tips.

- Use 100% cotton bedding.
- Avoid using duvets because they cause overheating (and eczema sufferers heat up quickly).
- Use woolen "breathable" blankets over cotton sheets in winter (but don't let woolen blankets touch the skin because they can cause irritation).
- Ensure cotton sheets are long so they completely cover blankets.

Clothing

- Take off tags from clothing because they can irritate the skin.
- Dress in 100% cotton clothing.
- Wear underclothing inside out so the seams are not irritating.

Laundry

- Change bed linens weekly.
- Wash sheets in hot water or use a dryer to kill the dust mites.
- Wash clothing in sensitive-skin or allergy washing powder and avoid fabric softeners.

Improve Your Sleeping Conditions

- Eczema sufferers benefit from having a sound night's sleep.
- Avoid overtiredness (go to bed early rather than late).

Did You Know?

Laughing Yourself to Sleep

Funny films are useful in treating nighttime waking in children with eczema, according to research by Dr. Hajime Kimata from the Department of Pediatrics and Allergy at the Ujitakeda Hospital in Kyoto, Japan. The benefit may be attributed in part to changes in the hormone level of ghrelin, which stimulates hunger. Compared to healthy children, salivary ghrelin levels are significantly elevated in patients with atopic eczema (which may make them feel hungry at bedtime or during the night). Research shows that viewing a humorous film before bedtime lowers salivary ghrelin levels and, as a result, children with eczema can experience a more restful night's sleep. Melatonin, the hormone that promotes proper sleep, is often lower in eczema sufferers compared with healthy people, and eczema sufferers can experience disturbed sleep as a result. Dr. Kimata reports that watching a funny film increases melatonin production. In breastfeeding women, laughter increases melatonin in their breast milk.

Dandruff, Seborrheic Dermatitis, and Cradle Cap

Dandruff and seborrheic dermatitis are flaking, itchy skin conditions that affect more than 50% of adults at some point in their life. With dandruff, the flakes are usually oily and shed easily from the scalp. Seborrheic dermatitis is a more severe skin condition with the addition of inflammation and greasy, yellowish flakes that can be found on the scalp, ears, eyebrows, neck, chest, and creases at the sides of the nose. Dandruff can occur when you have an oily scalp or if you are run down or stressed, and it can occur in conjunction with psoriasis and eczema. Newborn babies who develop cradle cap, which shows up as thick yellow crusts on the scalp, can develop dandruff later in life.

Although dandruff and seborrheic dermatitis appear when you have an oily scalp and altered microflora, these conditions do not occur on everyone.

Risk Factors

Susceptible people are at an increased risk of dandruff or seborrheic dermatitis because they have one or a combination of the following:

- Nutritional deficiencies and excess sugar and starch in the diet (sugar feeds fungus/yeasts)
- A predisposition to other skin conditions, such as cradle cap during childhood, psoriasis, or eczema
- Poor immunity (lowered defense against fungus, such as malassezia proliferation)
- Use of medical drugs
- Neurotransmitter abnormalities
- Damaged skin barrier/skin permeability (eczema!)
- Immune response and allergic reactions triggered by malassezia fungus/yeasts

Hair Care Practices

These hair care practices can affect the health of the scalp and increase the risk of dandruff:

- Hair product chemicals, such as sulfates, which are typically found in shampoos (see "Problematic Skin Care Products, page 128)
- Excess use of hair spray or gel
- Use of hair dyes
- Infrequent shampooing
- Inadequate rinsing of hair after washing
- pH changes in the scalp or skin (disrupted acid mantle or using hair-cleansing products that are alkaline)

Microflora Changes

The composition of scalp microflora is altered in people with dandruff and seborrheic dermatitis. Your immune system normally guards your skin from invading bacteria and yeasts, but when you're run down, stressed, or not feeding your body correctly, your immune system can let its guard down. A common yeast called malassezia (formerly called pityrosporum) lives on the scalp, and your immune system ensures that this freeloader doesn't multiply or claim too much territory. Research shows that 74% of the total microflora on the scalps of people with dandruff is malassezia and individuals with seborrheic dermatitis have 83% malassezia. In contrast, people with healthy scalps (no dandruff) have only 46% of the total microflora on their scalp as malassezia yeasts.

On healthy scalps, where there is no dandruff present, approximately 26% of the microflora is *Corynebacterium acnes*, a non-pathogenic bacteria, but it reduces to 6% in dandruff sufferers and to only 1% in seborrheic dermatitis patients.

> **Did You Know?**
> ....
> **Malassezia Yeasts**
> If your immune system fails to do its job, malassezia's "offspring, cousins, aunts, and uncles" take over your head and inflame your skin. Malassezia yeasts can be found on everyone, but they flourish and cause dandruff in approximately 20% of people.

Cradle Cap

Cradle cap is a form of scalp dermatitis. It is not caused by poor hygiene and it is not contagious. The sebaceous glands in the infant's skin become inflamed and produce excess oil, which traps the skin as it sheds, forming thick yellow crusts on the scalp. Cradle cap predominantly affects babies during their first few months of life; however, if untreated, it can persist until the age of 3 and, very rarely, beyond 3 years. Unlike eczema, cradle cap is not itchy and it does not usually cause babies discomfort. If a skin infection is suspected, see your doctor.

Guidelines for Managing Dandruff

There are three basic steps to treating and preventing dandruff.

Step 1: Swap your shampoo

Shampoos can alter the pH of the scalp, as can the use of gels, hair spray, and hair dyes. Swap your sulfate-containing shampoo for a gentle shampoo (note that some natural shampoos can aggravate dandruff, so you may need to try a few brands). There are a number of shampoo ingredients that are antifungal, antimicrobial, and anti-inflammatory, including:

- Tea tree oil
- Apple cider vinegar
- Vitamin E
- Panthenol (vitamin B_5)

In one study, patients with dandruff were given either a shampoo with 5% tea tree oil or a placebo shampoo. They were told to wash their hair daily, leaving the shampoo on for 3 minutes before rinsing. At the end of 4 weeks, scalp lesions were significantly lower and less itching was seen in the tea tree oil shampoo users.

Step 2: Spray your scalp

You can make this anti-dandruff remedy at home. This recipe is for the scalp only. Apply before bed. If desired, you can wash it off in the morning. Use a quality spray bottle because cheap plastic may buckle from the vinegar. You will need the following:

1	spray bottle	1
	Water	
½ tsp	tea tree oil	2 mL
16	drops pure vitamin E oil	16
2 tbsp	apple cider vinegar (not double strength)	30 mL

1. Fill the bottle with water.
2. Add the tea tree oil, vitamin E, and apple cider vinegar.
3. Close the lid and shake well.
4. Separate hair into sections so you can spray more directly onto the scalp. Spray your scalp.
5. Dry your hair and style as usual. Lightly spray onto the scalp once daily or as necessary.

Step 3: Eat a healthy diet

Follow the Eczema Diet to help promote a strong immune system. Parts 6 and 7 cover everything you need to know, including recipes, menus, and shopping guides, to get started on the Eczema Diet.

Symptoms of Cradle Cap

- Reddening of the skin
- Greasy scalp
- Thick yellow crusts that look like scabs/scales/flakes
- Mild discomfort
- Mild hair loss
- Inflammation with small blisters that eventually pop and weep
- Your child might be feeling ill

Causes of Cradle Cap

- Genetics (blood relatives are likely to have eczema and/or asthma)
- Overactive sebaceous glands (from maternal hormones)
- Appears in conjunction with seborrheic dermatitis (elsewhere on the body)

Cradle Cap Management

This is a two-step management plan for babies and children with cradle cap.

Step 1: Use gentle skin care

Hair: Find a natural baby shampoo that is free of sulfates (see "Problematic Skin Care Products," page 128). Be suspicious if a children's product foams and bubbles. Also avoid colored bath and skin products containing synthetic dyes and fragrances. You might need to visit your local health food shop to find a gentle baby shampoo (check the ingredients because some health food shops stock "natural" and "gentle" products that contain sodium lauryl sulfate). Shampoo your baby's hair and scalp often, but gently, to remove the cradle cap.

Body: Note that it is not essential to wash your baby's body with foaming cleansers or soaps, because this can disrupt the pH of their skin. Babies can be adequately cleaned with water and a very soft cloth.

Step 2: Use oil

Use a suitable oil to massage your baby's head — every second day if necessary (you can do this when you are bathing your baby). Then loosen the crusts by brushing the scalp, in a circular motion, with a very soft toothbrush, or you can gently use a plastic fine-tooth comb (not a metal one). Shampoo afterward to remove most of the oil.

Suitable Oils

To loosen the flakes, you can use the following oils:

- Calendula oil (diluted into a baby oil product)
- Flaxseed oil (can be used on its own)
- Evening primrose oil (can be used on its own)
- Natural vitamin E (diluted into a baby oil product)

First patch test the oil on unbroken skin and wait 24 hours to see if a reaction occurs. Do not use products containing mineral oil, and keep all oils out of children's reach.

Part 5

Children with Eczema

Chapter 7
Healthy Growth and Development

· ·

Testimonial

Clare has gone from vomiting up to 10 times daily to just once a week. She hasn't had any rashes for at least a fortnight. Clare stopped vomiting within 3 to 4 days after starting the diet and supplements. Her twin sister, Reese, is also a "new" baby girl... She's gone from a grumpy whiner to a happy little girl in the last few weeks. I am keeping the "new" baby! Reese's personality change happened about 10 days to 2 weeks after starting the new diet.

Jenny Bangor

Although eczema can occur at any age, it typically appears shortly after birth, between 2 and 6 months of age. More than half of all eczema sufferers show signs of eczema before their first birthday. As a parent, you will want to relieve your child from the aggravating and painful symptoms of eczema as soon as possible and ensure healthy growth and development long term.

The health and family history of an eczema sufferer, even of a newborn baby, can highlight key problem areas, such as susceptibility to fungal infections, chemical exposures, consumption of raw egg white by the mother during pregnancy, and so on. This case study isolates many of these problems, which you may encounter with your child.

CASE STUDY
Oscar's Environment

Oscar developed eczema when he was 8 weeks old. When solids were introduced at 6 months of age, his eczema spread over his entire body, and the eczema on his face made him look as though he was badly burned. When the family history was taken, a number of environmental problems emerged:

- Oscar's family lived in an area where crops were regularly sprayed with pesticides.
- Oscar's mother had been treated with antibiotics and antifungals to manage an infection and *Candida albicans* overgrowth before having a natural birth.
- Oscar's mother, while pregnant, frequently ate raw egg white (as whole-egg mayonnaise and small amounts of raw cake mix when baking). His mother experienced dry, itchy skin during this time but no rash was present.
- Oscar's mother noticed he would regularly pull away and cried "like he was in pain" while breastfeeding.
- Oscar had been previously treated with topical antibiotics and oral steroids, which caused his eczema to worsen, and his skin also had white patches.
- While the family was on holidays, Oscar was briefly treated with cortisone cream, which initially helped his eczema, but then it worsened.

Oscar's Treatment Plan

With this information, a treatment plan was developed that relieved many of Oscar's environmental symptoms:

- When Oscar's mother stopped consuming dairy products and eggs, she noticed that her baby fed more peacefully, and his previously explosive stool, which happened at every diaper change, ceased being runny and green and normalized to once daily. This indicated a need for probiotic supplements and foods for gastrointestinal health. Oscar was treated for fungal infection (oral and topical) before starting the Eczema Diet program. Oscar and his mother were to resume taking a probiotic supplement containing *L. rhamnosus* GG. Oscar was to consume a few grains by mouth.
- Oscar's mother was asked to stop taking her breastfeeding multivitamin supplement and was prescribed a supplement to increase glycine, magnesium, biotin, quercetin, and vitamins C, D, and E in her breast milk. The nutrients were chosen to help Oscar's liver deal with the chemical pesticide load from his environment and to supply nutrients for his

mother's health during breastfeeding. Only the mother was to take the supplement because the baby received the nutrients secondhand through the breast milk.

- Oscar's mother also took flaxseed oil as an omega-3 supplement.
- Oscar's mother changed her diet to eczema-safe foods and she consumed low-salicylate alkalizing vegetable juices daily.
- Because Oscar had recently started solids, a range of eczema-safe vegetables was added to his solids routine. Then meat was to be introduced to help boost iron consumption.

Oscar's eczema improved, but it was still present on his face and legs. Because Oscar's eczema worsened with the introduction of baby rice cereal at 6 months of age, his mother took rice out of their diets, and 2 weeks later, Oscar's eczema completely cleared up from his face and legs. He is now eczema-free.

First-Line Care of Children with Eczema

1. Reduce the itch by using the emergency "itch busters" described in the preface.

   - Cold compress
   - Baking soda bath
   - Alkalizing drink
   - Nutrient supplements

2. Use prescribed medicated creams if needed.

3. If your child has a flare-up from a particular food, refer to the "Eczema-Safe Food Guidelines" (page 174) to see which ingredient might be causing a reaction.

4. Review the symptom questionnaires in Chapter 2, then compare your child's condition to the case history in this chapter so you can better understand your child's experience of eczema.

Healthy Nutrition

Your child's healthy growth and development need special dietary attention from infancy through adolescence. Eczema can disrupt growth and development if left untreated.

Breastfeeding

When you are breastfeeding, the nutrients from your diet pass into the breast milk, and then your child's body uses these nutrients for growth, repair, and maintenance. While you are breastfeeding, you can modify your diet to change the nutrient composition in your milk so it is rich in anti-inflammatory and histamine-lowering nutrients. For a short period of time (approximately 3 months), you can also avoid consuming the foods that are known to exacerbate eczema, but take the recommended eczema supplements. Note that your baby is not to be given these supplements directly (unless it is a suitable probiotic), and breastfeeding mothers are not to do the 3-Day Alkalizing Cleanse or go hungry. Ensure you are consuming plenty of eczema-safe vegetables, protein, grains, vitamin C–rich papaya, and hydrating liquids. If you have a colicky or "windy" baby, you may also need to avoid garlic, leeks, and green onions.

Infant Formula

If your baby is drinking infant formula, speak to your pediatrician or doctor about changing your child to a low-allergy, non-dairy formula. Some probiotic supplements are suitable for infants. (See page 119 for more information on probiotics.)

Did You Know?

Sterilizing Your Baby's Water

For children under the age of 1 year, water must be boiled to sterilize and kill bacteria, and then cooled before giving it to your baby. Do not give pre-boiled water to infants after the age of 1, because your growing toddler's gastrointestinal tract needs to become accustomed to unsterilized water to challenge and strengthen the immune system. After the age of 1, regular filtered water (or filtered tap water) is recommended.

Starting Solids

"Solids" is the term used for the first foods you feed your baby. These foods are mushy and puréed to a smooth paste, not solid, as the word suggests. Recent research shows that delaying the introduction of solids for more than 6 months can increase the risk of allergy and eczema, so the current recommendation is to start your baby on solids after 4 months of age, unless advised otherwise by your pediatrician or doctor.

This general recommendation may not be suitable for all babies. Your baby needs to be able to sit upright while eating. If your baby is not showing signs of being ready for solids, you can delay introducing them for up to 6 months. Avoid serving foods that they can choke on, such as nuts, biscuits, toast, and solid pieces of fruit or vegetables. Sometimes babies have an adverse reaction to a new food they have tried, and diarrhea or vomiting is the result. Diarrhea and vomiting can cause dehydration and hydrating electrolytes may be required. Seek your doctor's advice if this occurs.

Testing for Child Food Allergies

To identify allergies and intolerances, introduce each new food on its own and then continue with that food for 3 days before introducing the next food. It is a good idea to introduce new foods earlier in the day, rather than at bedtime. Once your baby is in bed, you can't see if she is having an adverse reaction. If you introduce foods earlier in the day and your child has a life-threatening anaphylactic reaction, where they have swelling and difficulty breathing, you can spot it early and seek medical advice from a hospital or doctor. If your baby has a milder adverse reaction, such as a flare-up, unsettled behavior, diarrhea, or vomiting, keep a record in a diet diary and discontinue use of that particular food. You may want to re-test the food when your child is older.

Foods from 4 months

Continue to feed your baby breast milk or infant formula as usual. Then introduce the first food. In order of preference, these are:

1. **Plain baby rice cereal.** Ensure that the cereal is fortified with iron because your baby's iron stores begin to wane at this age. Choose plain varieties, no fruit flavors, and follow the packet instructions. If eczema symptoms worsen, discontinue use and seek advice from a nutritionist. Quinoa may be a suitable alternative, but note it does not contain added iron.

> **Did You Know?**
> ....
> ### Commercial Baby Foods
> Canned or jarred baby foods are generally not recommended because they may contain ingredients that make eczema symptoms worse; however, if it is a plain variety (e.g., plain potato or plain stewed pear), then it may be suitable on occasion or as a backup option. If using commercial baby food, check that all ingredients are eczema-safe.

2. **Puréed vegetables.** Eczema-safe vegetables are the best ones to try first. These include puréed white potato, sweet potato, and carrot (see "Stage 1 and Stage 2 Safe Foods Guide," page 91). If your child reacts to sweet potato or carrot, she may be sensitive to salicylates.

3. **Puréed fruit.** Don't give your baby fruit before vegetables because she may develop a sweet tooth and reject savory foods. Eczema-healthy fruits include peeled puréed pear, mashed banana (not sugar variety) and papaya. If your child reacts to banana or papaya, she may be sensitive to amines.

It is essential that your baby consume eczema-safe vegetables on a daily basis. Vegetables will help your child to be eczema-free.

Foods from 6 months

1. Continue to give your baby rice cereal, eczema-safe vegetables and fruit, and breast milk or infant formula during this time.

2. Add iron-rich meat or legumes to your baby's feeding routine because babies need extra iron in their diet for proper growth. When serving a baby meat, ensure the meat is very finely ground up. Start with lean lamb, followed by skinless chicken, both freshly ground. Preservative-free, antibiotic-free, free-range, organic, and fresh meat is best. Do not give your baby liver or other organ meat that can contain accumulated pesticides and chemicals.

3. Add mushy lentils, mashed chickpeas, mashed kidney beans, and so on (see "Stage 1 and Stage 2 Safe Foods Guide," page 91).

Foods from 8 months

1. If your baby is feeding well and ready for finger foods, give her small slices of soft eczema-safe fruits, steamed soft carrot sticks, sweet potato, and potato slices, and gluten-free rice or buckwheat pasta spirals.

2. Do not serve wheat pastas at this stage, and no long spaghetti.

Foods from 12 months

Your child should be consuming chopped-up foods by now, to experience different textures and flavors. Refer to Chapter 10 for a list of children's menu plans.

Foods to Avoid

Speak to your doctor about allergy testing. Fruit juice, cordial, and sodas are not recommended for babies. Avoid giving your baby other potentially problematic foods:

- Dairy products (cheese, yogurt, butter, cow's milk)
- Eggs
- Fish
- Peanut butter
- Tree nuts
- Sesame seeds (including tahini and sesame seed paste)

General Guidelines

Serving Sizes

How much is a serving? This table is designed to help you determine how many servings of each food group your child should be eating every day, depending on his age.

Age Group	Vegetables	Fruit	Grains	Non-Dairy Milk	Protein
1–3 years	1 to 2 servings ½ to 1 cup (125 to 250 mL)	1 to 2 servings ½ to 1 cup (125 to 250 mL)	1 to 2 servings ½ to 1 cup (125 to 250 mL)	1 to 2 servings ½ to 1 cup (125 to 250 mL)	1 to 2 servings ¼ to ½ cup (60 to 125 mL)
4–7 years	2 to 3 servings 1 to 1½ cups (250 to 375 mL)	2 servings 1 cup (250 mL)	2 servings 1 cup (250 mL)	2 servings 1 cup (250 mL)	1 serving ½ cup (125 mL)
8–17 years	3 to 4 servings 1½ to 2 cups (375 to 500 mL)	2 to 3 servings 1 to 1½ cups (250 to 375 mL)	2 to 3 servings 1 to 1½ cups (250 to 375 mL)	2 to 3 servings 1 to 1½ cups (250 to 375 mL)	1 to 2 servings ½ to 1 cup (125 to 250 mL)

Food Groups

If your child eats these servings from the major food groups on a daily basis, she should remain healthy and be able to combat eczema.

Vegetables: iceberg lettuce, romaine lettuce, mung bean sprouts, celery, cabbage (white or red), green beans, green onions, potatoes (but not russets), sweet potato, carrots, rutabaga (turnip), beets (fresh, not canned), parsley, chives, garlic (not Chinese), Brussels sprouts, and leeks.

Fruits: peeled pear, banana (not sugar variety), and papaya (the last two contain amines).

Grains: whole-grain oats, rice, spelt, barley, quinoa, and buckwheat, which are gluten-free.

Non-dairy milk: children with eczema should not consume dairy products, so it is necessary to get their calcium from non-dairy sources, such as rice milk and calcium-rich broths, which can be sipped warm during snack time or added to meals with mashed potato and casseroles.

Protein: protein foods contain iron, which is needed for healthy skin.

Guidelines for Treating Children with Eczema

1. Make your child as comfortable as possible using their prescribed medicated creams if necessary.
2. Select eczema-healthy foods from the Stage 1 shopping list (page 91) to prepare for meals and snacks. Photocopy this list and post it in your kitchen on a bulletin board or on the fridge. Take this list with you when you go shopping.
3. Serve your child appropriately sized amounts of food from the various food groups.
4. Use a diet diary to identify problematic foods and beneficial meals so you can tailor the program to suit your child.
5. Encourage the whole family to enjoy the eczema-healthy recipes. When families share meals, this can help the child with eczema feel normal and the all-important compliance with the Eczema Diet program is more likely.

Party Food Guide

Although party food generally causes itchy skin and a worsening of symptoms, it is possible to have an eczema-safe birthday party or other occasional celebration for your child. Here is a guide to party food for adults and children over 1 year old. These items are suggestions to choose from — you don't need to serve all of the foods listed. Ensure you choose items to suit the age of the partygoer, their possible food allergies, and feeding abilities. For example, a 1-year-old child may not be able to eat hard foods, such as toffee, and if someone is allergic to tree nuts, it is best to avoid serving them. Check with the parents of each child you invite.

Party Foods

Refer to the recipes section of this book for eczema-safe treats you can create for your child's party.

Eczema-Safe Packaged Party Foods	Eczema-Safe Homemade Foods
Children	
Lemonade, bottled (no colors or preservatives)	Filtered water
Natural mineral water (no flavors or colors)	Birthday Cake (page 248)
Soda water	Cupcakes (from Birthday Cake recipe)
Lemonade ice pops (plain only; no colors or preservatives)	Baked Banana Chips (page 242)
Potato chips and french fries (plain or salted only; no color, flavor enhancers, or additives)	Carrot and celery sticks served with Parsley Pesto (page 241) (contains cashews) or Sesame-Free Hummus (page 239)
Mini packets of plain potato chips	Potato Wedges (page 233), served warm
Rice crackers (plain or salted only; no flavor enhancers, additives, or corn)	New Anzac Cookies (page 250)
Green soybeans (edamame)	Papaya Rice Paper Rolls (page 222)
Caramels, plain (no additives) Toffee, plain (no additives) White marshmallows	Spelt Chips (variation, page 243), served with Sesame-Free Hummus (page 239)
Honeycomb	
Adults only	
Gin Tonic water, bottled (no preservatives) Vodka and soda Whisky and soda	Decaffeinated coffee (with soy milk) Unsalted cashews

Party Treat Bags

Children usually like to have goodie bags of sweets given to them at the end of a party. Many of the eczema-safe party foods will help fill a treat bag, as will kids' bracelets, cheap jewelry, homemade beaded items, balloons, whistles, mini plastic dinosaurs, and other small figurines from a discount shop or dollar store. Here are some suggestions for eczema-safe treat bags.

Goodie Bag 1
- Caramels (plain; no additives or chocolate)
- White marshmallows
- Plastic bracelet or figurine
- Balloon
- Whistle or mini bubble blower (if not sensitive to dishwashing liquid)

Goodie Bag 2
- Eczema-safe cupcake with plain icing, wrapped in clear or colored cellophane, and tied with a colorful ribbon
- Stickers

Goodie Bag 3
- White marshmallows
- Honeycomb
- Balloon
- Stickers

Treat Days

If you would like to treat yourself or your child occasionally, set strict guidelines. If you stick to these guidelines, it should not affect your results (but might delay them slightly).

1. Choose only treats from the list of eczema-safe treats in this chapter.

2. Set a specific day and time when you can enjoy a treat. For example, "Treat day is Sunday," when you can have pure maple syrup on pancakes for breakfast (using eczema-safe ingredients), a couple of marshmallows after lunch or dinner, and Chocolate Milk (page 210) after dinner or as a morning snack. Other examples include "Ice pop day is Friday" (use plain lemonade). Adults can set limits as well, such as "I can drink alcohol at birthday parties and weddings" (2 glasses or less of eczema-safe alcohol every 2 weeks). If you are craving sweet foods or alcohol, see "Sugar Cravings" (page 74) for ways to reduce these desires.

Did You Know?

The Truth about Sugar

Although unhealthy sugar-rich and fried foods are listed as eczema-safe in this chapter, avoid these foods on a daily or regular basis. Most of these eczema-safe party foods and drinks are considered unhealthy because they take more nutrients to process than they supply, thereby depleting the body of valuable nutrients needed for healthy skin. Furthermore, sugary foods increase acid in the body, so they may exacerbate the itch.

To help counteract the negative effects from eating sugar-rich or fried foods, drink a glass of highly alkalizing juice, such as Tarzan Juice (page 207) or Healthy Skin Juice (page 206), or eat an Alkaline Bomb Salad (page 218). You could also add mung bean sprouts to your next meal to help restore your acid-alkaline balance.

Chapter 8
Children's Special Needs

● ●

Testimonial

I have been recently trying your advice about giving my 5-year-old, who suffers terribly from eczema, a daily dose of the supplement for salicylate sensitivity. I must say that after 3 days, his skin is beautiful. I have never seen it look this good. Combined with your diet, I am so grateful for a different child.

Cathi Firth

One in five children has eczema and, according to the National Eczema Society in the United Kingdom, there are no guarantees that a child will grow out of eczema, although approximately 74% are eczema-free by the age of 16. However, dietary changes can markedly speed up this process, especially if parents and caregivers attend to their children's special dietary needs. The following case history isolates a few of these needs.

Q. Our family is vegetarian. Must my daughter eat meat if she has eczema?

A. If you are vegetarian or vegan, it is not necessary to eat red meat, fish, or chicken during the Eczema Diet. Recipes containing meat are on the menu to supply protein and iron. To meet protein and iron requirements, choose vegetarian soups and eat beans if preferred. Several vegan and vegetarian options are given in the recipe section of this book. Many of the recipes in the menus are already suitable for vegetarians and vegans. Avoid these foods: tempeh, vegan/vegetarian patties and sausages, and other meat substitutes; they can contain additives, soy sauce, flavorings, and herbs that could make the eczema flare up.

CASE STUDY
Riley's Environment

By the time he was 15 months old, Riley's eczema had spread to most of his body. A complete health history was taken, which revealed some precipitating causes:

- Riley had acid reflux for the first 6 months of life, which indicates he would benefit from alkalizing foods in the diet, such as eczema-safe vegetables, bananas, and magnesium, to promote acid-alkaline balance each day.
- Riley has suffered from eczema since he was 3 months old.
- Both his parents have hay fever, and his aunt and uncle have asthma.
- Riley's eczema periodically worsens if there is any change in routine, if he visits the family farm, where pesticides are used, and if he eats specific foods.
- The problematic foods in Riley's diet are watermelon, mangos, avocados, melon, passion fruit, mandarins, strawberries, jam, popcorn, margarine (high in omega-6 fatty acids), olive oil, broccoli, spaghetti bolognese (tomato), corn and corn pasta, and baked beans, which are rich in salicylates and natural MSG.
- Riley's eczema visibly worsens on hot and humid days, after swimming in chlorinated pools, after contact with grass or when crawling on carpet, during sudden weather changes, on windy days, and from stress.
- He always flares up for 2 weeks after receiving immunizations, which suggests his body may be slow at eliminating histamine from the blood (indicating the need for supplemental vitamin C, vitamin B_6, and quercetin, and papaya in the diet). He has been tested for allergies and is allergic to dairy, eggs, wheat, codfish (other fish are okay), nuts, sesame seeds, latex, and rye grass.
- He has shown no signs of fungal infection or candida overgrowth.
- Riley's mother ate raw egg white (whole-egg mayonnaise and hollandaise sauce) once a month before, but not during, pregnancy.
- His mother was managing Riley's eczema by moisturizing him throughout the day, and he was given an antihistamine before bed if he was itchy. Topical steroids were applied on the red patches.
- Riley's mother had already taken steps to make the house eczema-safe: she was ventilating the house daily and was already giving her child a suitable probiotic supplement for eczema.

continued...

Riley's Treatment Plan

- His mother was advised to avoid the problematic foods and was given eczema-safe shopping lists, recipes, and menus.
- A supplement was prescribed for Riley, which included biotin, glycine, magnesium, vitamin C, natural vitamin E, vitamin B12, folic acid, vitamin B6, zinc, alpha-lipoic acid, quercetin, vitamin K, vitamin D3, chromium, choline, inositol, and calcium.
- Three months after the initial consultation, Riley is walking. His eczema does not flare up from carpet contact, and changes in routine are not really a problem now. Within about 2 weeks of starting the Eczema Diet, Riley's skin improved. His skin continues to improve and remains clearer for longer. He no longer has all-over-body red rashes.
- His mother still steers clear of foods that cause allergic reactions, but she has reintroduced some of these foods in moderation (once a week) and he seems to be fine with that.

Supplemental Iron

A child should eat 2 servings of protein foods containing iron each day for healthy growth and development. Iron deficiency can cause anemia and slow growth.

Iron Sources

Iron sources from richest to poorest are:

- Red meat
- Commercial rice or oat cereals with added iron
- Beans
- Lentils
- Whole wheat pasta
- Tofu
- Chicken
- Fish
- Whole wheat bread

When you give your child a serving of iron-rich food, be sure not to serve calcium-rich foods at the same time. Calcium can prevent iron absorption. A child aged 1 to 3 years needs 9 mg of iron daily, which is equivalent to 2 servings of protein-rich foods.

Vaccinations

Vaccinating your child is a personal choice, but if your child has eczema, here are some facts to consider:

- Catching measles or having vaccinations for measles, mumps, and rubella (MMR) can trigger the appearance of atopic dermatitis, according to several research studies. This may be related to nutritional deficiencies, such as vitamin C. Studies show that vitamin C is depleted after receiving vaccinations, causing blood histamine levels to markedly increase, which can cause adverse symptoms. Taking vitamin C before and after vaccinations may assist with recovery, and babies on solids can be fed vitamin C–rich papaya.
- Some vaccines, such as MMR vaccines and the flu vaccine, contain traces of egg, so if your child has an allergy to egg, mention this to your doctor so that you might opt for an egg-free alternative.

Some doctors advise delaying immunizations if a child is unwell or has atopic eczema. If you are concerned about vaccinating your child, please seek further information from your doctor. Immunizations can and do save lives when outbreaks occur.

Q. What is the first thing I should feed my child after his immunizations?

A. Before and after your child has vaccinations, feed him papaya. Blood histamine levels elevate after immunizations, which can make him appear unwell, and papaya is a rich source of histamine-lowering vitamin C. If you are breastfeeding, ensure you are taking vitamin C, quercetin, and vitamin B6, because they will pass through the breast milk and can help your baby deal with the histamine influx caused by immunizations.

Teething

Teething Problems

If your baby is teething, you can make homemade rice rusks that are wheat- and dairy-free. They are easy to make. See the recipe on page 204.

Teething Gels

Avoid teething gels because they are rich in salicylates and can cause severe flare-ups in sensitive children. If you have a baby with eczema who is teething, you have a couple of options:

1. Use teething toys, such as a freezeable teething ring, which can be placed in the freezer and given to your child to chew on when the ring is cold.
2. If your child needs pain relief, talk to your doctor about using color-free baby acetaminophen. Rub a very small amount onto your child's gums if she is unsettled because of teething pain.

Fussy Eating Habits

Some children are fussy eaters. They reject certain foods, scream when you try to feed them new foods, and generally make eating a chore. To address this problem, slogans have been added to the recipes in this book, such as "Time for eczema-safe veggies" and "Morning tea is fruit time." These phrases are effective tools to help guide a young child to accept and enjoy a healthy eating program. If said daily, these phrases can help your child form new eating habits over a matter of days or weeks.

Rate Your Child's Eczema

Before beginning the Eczema Diet program, try rating the severity of your child's eczema on a scale of 1 (best) to 10 (worst). Take photos of your child's eczema so you can compare symptoms before and after. You will be surprised by the result.

Start/End Date	Skin Condition
Start Date: _____	/10 Description:
End Date: _____	/10 Description:

CASE HISTORY
Hopeless Case

Dietary therapy for children's eczema is not new. In the *British Medical Journal* back in 1882, a doctor described a diet that rapidly cured his eczema-afflicted patients. He documented a particularly "hopeless case" of a 9-year-old boy who had suffered from eczema since he was 5 months old. The child had been under constant medical care, in and out of hospitals for more than 8 years, and no prescribed treatment, cream, or drug had ever improved his eczema. When he was admitted to hospital for eczema treatment on this occasion, the doctor placed the child on a modified diet. The diet was low in fat, dairy-free, and sugar-free. All fat was cut off meats, and poultry was recommended instead of pork. An oil supplement was prescribed. Beef broth was given, with the fat carefully skimmed off, and he ate baked fish, not fried. Within a fortnight, the child's skin showed improvement, and a month later, his eczema was practically gone and he was discharged from hospital.

Part 6

Planning the Eczema Diet

Chapter 9
Stocking Up and Starting Out

· ·

Testimonial

The diet plus all the supplements worked so well for us. I felt like a miracle happened to Leo. (He had regular steroid creams from a very early age, on top of antibiotics for infections on the skin that often happened because of various reasons, including childcare and very itchy nights.) We had flaxseed oil and probiotics and other natural supplements before, but I think the combination and diet that you described is the most effective. (I also learned a lot for myself, for my own health! Many thanks for this too.) My younger one also has a bit of eczema, but just a few spots, which is such a relief! When we did the diet, we had it pretty much for the whole family. Milan's eczema also completely disappeared.

Natalya L.

If **you are** well prepared, the Eczema Diet is not difficult to implement and maintain. You will need to do some shopping for food and perhaps a few cooking utensils, depending on how well your pantry, cupboards, and refrigerator are stocked. Get everything lined up before you start to prepare meals following the 14-day menu plans and the recipes provided. Once you have mastered Stage 1 and your eczema has begun to heal, you can add more foods to your diet following the Stage 2 and Stage 3 food guidelines presented in this chapter.

Taking Stock
Peek in the Pantry

Read ahead to the menu plans and recipes and refer to the
"Stage 1 Safe Foods Guide" (page 91) while compiling your
shopping list. For future reference, you could photocopy that
guide and post it on your refrigerator door or on a bulletin
board. Check off food items and ingredients that you already
have in stock. You may need some help from the staff at your
local health food store to track down a few of the more exotic
food items.

Check Your Appliances and Utensils

Here is a list of the basic needed kitchen tools you likely already
have in your kitchen:

- Beater
- Graters
- Measuring cups and spoons
- Basting and pastry brushes
- Muffin pan
- Large baking sheet
- Saucepans
- Frying pans: large and small nonstick frying pans
- Casserole and baking dishes: a large casserole and a
  roasting pan with a lid

Here is a list of a few new tools that may also come in handy:

- **Salad spinner:** works well to "dry" vegetables after
  washing them to remove any contaminants
- **Water filter jug:** no need to install expensive water filters
  unless you want to
- **Food processor:** mixes muffins, grates vegetables, and
  whips up tasty dips
- **Juicer:** makes fresh vegetable juices and speeds up results;
  a juicer can speed up skin recovery time, although eczema
  patients have healed without the addition of juices, so you
  may be fine without one
- **Slow cooker:** makes soups, broth, and casseroles, though
  it is not essential to have one

Making Stock

You will make your life easier if you prepare a few things 1 or 2 days before you begin the diet. Therapeutic Broth (page 212) is a key recipe throughout this diet and you will need to allocate time to let it simmer and gather richness (6 hours or more). Then you need to let it cool down overnight in the refrigerator so it is easy to remove all the fat from the top. If the fat is not totally removed, it will sabotage your diet; don't skip this step. The broth will stay fresh for up to 6 days, so you may need to freeze the leftovers.

It is handy to freeze 1-tablespoon (15 mL) portions in an ice cube tray, covered in plastic wrap. Then you can run the back of the tray under hot water to release them when you require them in a recipe for your child's dinner, for example. The soups and casseroles all require 3 cups (750 mL) of Therapeutic Broth, so you can freeze portions of 3 cups (750 mL) of broth in freezer-proof containers for later use (though if you are an adult doing the 3-Day Alkalizing Cleanse, you will use up the broth within the 3 days).

Other Useful Recipes

If you have a child with eczema, you might want to bake some muffins for your child's lunch box (page 203) and make Sesame-Free Hummus (page 239). These two recipes are not essential to the diet but they are handy. Also soak some oats or quinoa grains at the end of day 3 in preparation for breakfast on day 4. For breakfast on day 4, make Omega Muesli (page 198), or if you are gluten intolerant, try Quinoa Porridge (page 200).

Starting Stage 1
Prepare for the 3-Day Alkalizing Cleanse

Adults with eczema are advised to do the 3-Day Alkalizing Cleanse. Start by writing down the ingredients for these recipes. You will need to buy your supplements before you begin the cleanse. The cleanse is not suitable for children, pregnant or breastfeeding women, or anyone who has a medical condition requiring medical drugs.

Did You Know?

Food-Based Cleanse

The 3-Day Alkalizing Cleanse is a highly nutritious and gentle food-based cleanse that is gluten-free, low in natural chemicals, and contains no artificial chemicals.

Recipes for the 3-Day Alkalizing Cleanse

- Therapeutic Broth, page 212
- Alkaline Veggie Broth, page 214 (alternative broth for vegetarians and vegans)
- New Potato and Leek Soup, page 215
- Chickpea Casserole, page 224
- Tarzan Juice, page 207

Foods to Enhance the Cleanse

- Enhance Phase 2 liver detoxification by cooking with fresh garlic and eat either cabbage or Brussels sprouts daily (these are included in the recipes).
- Drink filtered water, 5 to 8 glasses (48 to 64 ounces, or 1.5 to 2 L) daily.
- Eat these raw veggies daily: celery, mung bean sprouts, green onions, iceberg lettuce (don't eat other raw veggies during the cleanse).
- If needed, also eat the following steamed veggies: cabbage, green beans, Brussels sprouts, white potato.
- Use chives and parsley as flavoring.

Cleansing Tips

- Don't go hungry: eat as much soup, casserole, and/or raw veggies as you like, and drink plenty of Tarzan Juice (at least 2 servings).
- Don't go out socializing during the cleanse, because you need to rest and to avoid all other foods and drinks for 3 days.
- Take eczema-safe supplements, including vitamin C (plus vitamin K), glycine, vitamin B6, magnesium, natural vitamin E, biotin, zinc, alpha-lipoic acid, quercetin, vitamin D3, and chromium, to stay nourished and to help speed up results.

Starting Stage 2

Waiting until your eczema has completely healed before moving on to Stage 2 is recommended. The only reason to move ahead to Stage 2 at a faster pace would be if you had to increase the range of foods in your diet due to boredom or fussy eating habits and you were happy to risk slowing down your results. (On saying this, you may find Stage 2 foods don't cause any adverse reactions, so you can happily expand your diet.)

Q. When do I begin Stage 2?

A. It's up to you to decide when you begin Stage 2. Be aware that rushing into Stage 2 prematurely can set you back and may affect your results. The following are basic guidelines for moving on to Stage 2:

1. Your eczema should be visibly improving and your skin should be holding moisture better. It is a good sign if you can start using a lighter moisturizer and your skin is showing signs of healing and is not flared up.
2. Your eczema should be consistently improving. If you are still having random, unexplained flare-ups, you need to do some additional investigation to identify what you are reacting to (and then stop exposing yourself to it).
3. You need to be happy with your results before moving on to Stage 2.

Stage 2 is the second part of the Eczema Diet, where you can introduce other types of foods, along with Stage 1 ingredients. This is an important step to increase the variety of foods in your diet and this stage can also help you identify food sensitivities. Particular foods have been selected for Stage 2 because they add extra nutrients and flavors to the diet.

Tomato Caution

Tomato is traditionally problematic for eczema sufferers because it is rich in natural MSG, which gives tomato products their lovely flavor. Raw tomato may be the most problematic, so eat cooked tomato and only in moderation.

Stage 2 Vegetables

All vegetables are alkalizing, so it is important to expand your range as soon as possible. Try one new food every 3 days and note any adverse reactions in your diet diary. If an adverse reaction occurs, discontinue use and re-test the food in 2 months' time if desired. Add these "moderate" salicylate vegetables and herbs into your diet:

- Asparagus
- Bok choy
- Basil
- Chicory
- Cilantro
- Endive
- Mint
- Peas (fresh or frozen) (they contain natural MSG)
- Snow peas
- Snow pea sprouts
- Baby squash
- Turnip
- Yam

Organic Tomato Sauce

Tomato is an important part of Stage 2 because it is rich in skin-protective lycopene. The most powerful antioxidant of all the carotenoids, lycopene can reduce the risk of skin cancer and prostate cancer, and, if consumed regularly, it has a mild protective effect against sunburn. Cooked tomato contains more lycopene than raw.

Plain organic tomato sauce has been chosen for Stage 2 because it is pleasant for all ages to consume (especially children) and it should have no artificial additives. It is an optional addition to your diet if you miss using sauce. Begin with 1 teaspoon (5 mL) once or twice weekly (a maximum of 1 teaspoon/5 mL for children and 2 teaspoons/10 mL for adults, up to three times weekly). If you have an adverse reaction to tomato sauce, discontinue use. Alternatively, you can eat a slice of papaya daily to ensure you consume lycopene in the diet (this is most important).

Q. Must I eat meat?

A. Please note it is not necessary to eat red meat, fish, or chicken during the Eczema Diet. Recipes containing meat are in the menu mainly for variety (and they supply protein and iron). Please choose vegetarian soups and eat beans if preferred.

Q. I'm a vegetarian. What can I eat from the Eczema Diet?

A. Eczema-safe vegetarian protein sources are chickpeas, green beans, raw cashews (if no nut allergy), tofu, lentils, kidney beans, and other beans (but not fava beans). Many of the recipes in the menus are already suitable for vegetarians and vegans, and most recipes can be converted so they are suitable for vegetarians and vegans, with the exception of Easy Roast Chicken, Baked Fish with Mash, and Therapeutic Broth (Alkaline Veggie Broth, page 214, is a suitable broth alternative). If a dinner recipe contains an animal product that cannot be substituted, try a soup option.

Onions

White and red onions are rich in the flavonoid quercetin, so onions can make a nutritious addition to your diet. Onions are high in salicylates, however, so try the other Stage 2 vegetables first, and if no adverse reactions occur, you may like to test onions (eating onions in the diet is optional). Discontinue use if you have an adverse reaction to them.

All other vegetables, such as spinach and broccoli, are very high in salicylates and other natural chemicals, so do not eat them just yet. You can expand your vegetable range further once Stage 2 vegetables have passed the test.

Stage 2 Fruits

Stage 2 fruits contain "moderate" salicylates and they have been chosen because they are highly nutritious. Note that blueberries and lemons are high in salicylates (lemon also contains lots of amines), but they have been chosen for Stage 2 because of their rich antioxidant content and for lemon's strong alkalizing effect; and watermelon contains lycopene. Add these salicylate fruits into your diet (one every 3 days if desired):

- Apples, Golden Delicious and Red Delicious (other varieties are high in salicylates)
- Watermelon
- Blueberries
- Lime
- Lemon (test lemon last)

How to Test Lemon

First test the other fruits, such as Red Delicious apples, watermelon, and blueberries. If they all pass the test (and your eczema does not return), then consume 1 teaspoon (5 mL) of lemon juice daily for 1 to 3 days. If no reaction occurs, try Flaxseed Lemon Drink (page 208). Lemon is useful for flavoring fish and pasta recipes, and Flaxseed Lemon Drink is fantastic for the skin (if you don't have an adverse reaction to the lemon). If an adverse reaction occurs, note it in your diet diary, discontinue use, and re-test lemon in 1 to 2 months' time if desired.

Stage 2 Spices and Herbs

Spices and herbs offer you an impressive range of flavonoids, antioxidants, and delicious flavours that can make a diet rich and interesting. Cinnamon and cumin are two of the most valuable spices for eczema sufferers. Cinnamon and cumin contain high salicylates, but they can be used in small amounts. If these ones don't cause flare-ups, you can try other spices, such as whole nutmeg (grated onto porridge). One range of spices you may have ongoing problems with is curry powder, because it is incredibly rich in salicylates, so don't try curry just yet. Basil and mixed herbs can be used in casseroles, and dried mint flakes enhance lamb.

Cinnamon

Cinnamon plays a starring role in Stage 2 because this delicious spice contains cinnamaldehyde, which lowers blood glucose level and slows the absorption of carbohydrates in the intestines. To test it, add a sprinkling of cinnamon to Omega Muesli (page 198), Quinoa Porridge (page 200), or Surprise Porridge (page 199) and then see if there are any adverse reactions in the 3 days that follow. If an adverse reaction occurs, note it in your diet diary, discontinue use, and re-test cinnamon in 1 to 2 months' time. Continue taking a chromium supplement because chromium also improves blood glucose tolerance.

If there is no adverse reaction, you can add it to foods such as Cinnamon Chicken (page 227) or sprinkle it onto potatoes before baking to help lower your blood insulin level (which can spike after eating potato and carbohydrate-rich grains).

Ground Cumin

Cumin can decrease blood sugar and it contains antioxidants, which are beneficial for the heart. It makes recipes such as hummus, casseroles, and meat dishes taste delicious. Add a sprinkling of ground cumin to Sesame-Free Hummus (page 239), and if no adverse reaction occurs, add it to Chickpea Casserole (page 224) or sprinkle it onto Easy Roast Chicken (page 228).

Other Stage 2 Additions

You might like to try reintroducing the following alkalizing foods into your diet at this stage. Note that these three ingredients may cause adverse reactions. It is not essential to add these to your diet.

Organic Butter

This Stage 2 addition is optional. Do not use butter if you have an allergy to dairy products. Butter was chosen because pure organic butter contains no additives and it is slightly alkalizing when unheated. It is the least reactive of all the dairy products, so it may be well tolerated if you don't have an allergy to dairy products. Do not use butter for cooking, because the smoking point is too low. If an adverse reaction occurs, note it in your diet diary, discontinue use, and, if desired, re-test dairy products in 2 months' time. Because this product is rich in saturated fats, it is essential to keep butter use to a minimum.

Apple Cider Vinegar

Vinegar can be handy for making delicious salad dressings and this one has health benefits too. Although most vinegars are strongly acid-forming and unsuitable for eczema sufferers, apple cider vinegar is highly alkalizing and it can be beneficial for eczema. There is a catch, however. Apple cider vinegar is rich in natural chemicals, including sulfites, salicylates, and moderate amines, so it may cause your eczema to return, especially if you are sensitive to sulfites (if you have sulfite allergy, do not test apple cider vinegar).

If you do not have sulfite sensitivity, test apple cider vinegar in the delicious Omega Salad Dressing (page 220). Wait up to 3 days to see if there is an adverse reaction. If an adverse reaction occurs, note it in your diet diary and discontinue use. Alternatively, once this ingredient has passed the test, you can use the dressing on salads, such as Alkaline Bomb Salad (page 218) and Roasted Sweet Potato Salad (page 219). Apple cider vinegar has potent antibacterial and preserving qualities, so you can use a splash in water to clean vegetables and sprouts.

Liquid Chlorophyll

Low-strength liquid chlorophyll (not high-strength) can be taken with chilled filtered water as a way to lower acidity in the body and ensure a healthy acid-alkaline balance to maintain clear skin (optional only). If an adverse reaction occurs, note it in your diet diary and discontinue use.

Adult dosage: begin with ½ teaspoon (2 mL) daily and work your way up to 1 to 2 teaspoons (5 to 10 mL) daily. Consult with your doctor before giving liquid chlorophyll to a child.

Q. Can I eat chia seeds during the Eczema Diet?

A. Chia seeds are tiny seeds that can be sprinkled onto breakfast cereals and porridge and they are becoming popular because of their omega-3 content. Gluten-free chia bread is also available from some health food shops. However, because they are a newly popular food with little scientific data available on them, we are unsure of their chemical composition so we cannot add them to the eczema-safe list at present. If you want to try them, add them to your diet during Stage 2, while your skin is clear, and see if you react to them. If your skin remains clear after 3 days, you can safely enjoy them. Flax seeds are an eczema-safe alternative (if you are not allergic to flax seeds).

Starting Stage 3

Stage 3 is an unofficial stage during which, if you would like to, you can add wheat and dairy back into your diet and see if you can tolerate them without your eczema returning. These foods should be limited.

Organic Plain Yogurt

If you have a child recovering from eczema, she has either totally forgotten about dairy products by now or is really, really missing them. Cow's milk (light and full-fat) often causes eczema to return in Stage 3, so you might want to delay introducing animal milks. Children can quickly become addicted to dairy products and their eczema can return. However, a small weekly, then daily, serving of quality organic yogurt can be well tolerated if your child is not allergic to dairy products. Look for these criteria when choosing yogurt:

- Must not contain natural annatto color 160b
- Must not contain artificial additives
- Must not contain added sugar

Plain organic and additive-free Greek yogurts are usually suitable; organic vanilla yogurt may also be suitable (if it contains no additives). You can sweeten plain yogurt with rice malt syrup, Banana Carob Spread (page 238), or eczema-safe fruits.

Did You Know?

Wheat Testing

When testing wheat, choose quality wheat products first, such as whole wheat sourdough bread. If an adverse reaction occurs, note it in your diet diary, discontinue use, and re-test the food in 1 to 2 months' time if desired.

Eczema-Safe Food Guidelines

This list of common foods is designed to show you what foods to eat when you have eczema and what foods to avoid. Each food is categorized by food group and analyzed for pH (alkalinity and acidity), salicylates, sulfites, amines, additives, glycemic index, and gluten content. These are the chemicals most important in the onset of eczema and your recovery. Here is how the guidelines work.

At a quick glance, you can see that, for example, broccoli is strongly alkalizing but contains high salicylates, amines, and MSG (natural monosodium glutamate). Each of these chemicals can trigger eczema flare-ups, so broccoli should be avoided. However, you can also see that carrots are alkalizing, with no sulfites and only moderate salicylate content. For this reason, carrots are eczema-safe. Although broccoli should be avoided while you are following Stage 1 of the Eczema Diet, it can be slowly re-introduced to your list of healthy foods as you recover in Stage 2 and Stage 3.

How do you make the decision whether to eat or avoid a food on this list? I have taken the guesswork out of the process by **bolding** eczema-safe foods. Stock up on these foods the next time you go shopping. These foods are used extensively in the recipe section of this book.

The guidelines are particularly useful if you have identified a food that causes your eczema to flare up. For example, if you react to dried figs, you can look at the fruit section of the list and see that dates, raisins, and other dried fruit are all high in salicylates and sulfites. It would likely be best if you avoided these foods.

There are a number of non-allergy foods that can cause severe flare-ups; these are listed in the "Severe Reactions" column.

Continue to avoid foods and drinks you are allergic to and see an allergy specialist if you have not had your allergies formally diagnosed.

	Strongly Alkalizing	Alkalizing	Acidifying	Strongly Acidifying	Moderate Salicylates	Very High Salicylates	Sulfites	Amines	High Amines	MSG	High Glycemic Index	Gluten	Additives	Severe Reactions
CARBOHYDRATES: VEGETABLES														
Artichoke		•			•									
Arugula	•				•									
Asparagus		•		•										
Barley grass	•				•							•		•
Beets, raw	•			•										
Bell pepper		•			•									
Broccoli	•				•			•		•				
Brussels sprouts		•												
Cabbage, white & red		•												
Carrot		•		•										

	Strongly Alkalizing	Alkalizing	Acidifying	Strongly Acidifying	Moderate Salicylates	Very High Salicylates	Sulfites	Amines	High Amines	MSG	High Glycemic Index	Gluten	Additives	Severe Reactions
Cauliflower		•			•									
Celery		•												
Chicory		•		•										
Chinese greens		•		•										
Corn			•		•									
Dark leafy greens	•				•									
Eggplant (aubergine)		•			•			•						
Endive		•		•										
Gherkin (pickled)			•		•	•			•					
Green beans		•												
Green onion (scallions)		•												
Kale, raw	•				•									
Leek		•												
Lettuce, romaine		•		•										
Lettuce, iceberg		•												
Mushroom		•			•				•	•				
Olive		•			•				•					
Onion		•			•									
Parsnip		•		•							•			
Peas, fresh or frozen			•	•							•			
Peas, dried, cooked			•											
Pickled vegetables			•		•	•			•					•
Pumpkin (squash)		•		•							•			
Radish		•			•									
Rutabaga		•												
Swiss chard			•		•				•	•				
Snow pea		•		•										
Spinach, raw	•				•			•	•					
Sprouts, alfalfa	•				•									
Sprouts, lentil	•													
Sprouts, mung bean	•													
Sprouts, snow pea	•			•										
Squash, baby (pattypan)		•		•										
Squash, summer		•		•										

	Strongly Alkalizing	Alkalizing	Acidifying	Strongly Acidifying	Moderate Salicylates	Very High Salicylates	Sulfites	Amines	High Amines	MSG	High Glycemic Index	Gluten	Additives	Severe Reactions
Tomato, raw		●			●				●	●				
Tomato, cooked			●		●				●	●				
Turnip		●			●									
Yam		●			●									
Watercress	●				●									
Wheat grass juice	●				●									●
Zucchini		●			●									
CARBOHYDRATES: FRUIT														
Apples			●		●									
Apricot			●		●									
Avocado		●			●				●					
Banana (not sugar variety)		●						●						
Berries			●		●									
Black currant				●	●									
Blackthorn berry				●	●									
Cherries			●		●									
Date		●			●				●		●			
Dried fruit			●		●		●							
Figs			●		●		●		●					
Grapes			●		●				●	●				
Grapefruit	●				●				●					
Lemon	●				●				●					
Lime	●				●				●					
Mandarin				●	●				●					
Mango			●		●									
Mulberry				●	●									
Nectarine				●	●									
Orange				●	●				●					
Papaya			●					●						
Pears, peeled			●											
Persimmon			●		●									

	Strongly Alkalizing	Alkalizing	Acidifying	Strongly Acidifying	Moderate Salicylates	Very High Salicylates	Sulfites	Amines	High Amines	MSG	High Glycemic Index	Gluten	Additives	Severe Reactions
Pineapple			•		•				•					
Plum			•		•				•	•				
Pomegranate			•		•									
Kiwi			•		•				•					
Raisins		•			•				•	•				
Raspberry			•		•				•					
Strawberry			•		•									
Watermelon			•		•						•			

CARBOHYDRATES: GRAINS, FLOUR, BREADS

	Strongly Alkalizing	Alkalizing	Acidifying	Strongly Acidifying	Moderate Salicylates	Very High Salicylates	Sulfites	Amines	High Amines	MSG	High Glycemic Index	Gluten	Additives	Severe Reactions
Amaranth			•								•			
Baby rice cereal			•											
Barley			•									•		
Basmati rice			•											
Brown rice			•								•			
Buckwheat			•											
Corn			•		•									
Corn chips			•	•										
Corn flakes cereal			•		•						•			
Cornflour			•								•			
Corn cakes			•								•			
Couscous (semolina)			•								•	•		
Cracked wheat			•								•	•		
Millet			•								•			
Muesli			•			•		•						
Oats, rolled			•									•		
Oat milk			•								•	•		
Pasta (wheat)			•									•		
Polenta (cornmeal)			•		•						•			
Potato, new	•				•									
Potato, white	•										•			

	Strongly Alkalizing	Alkalizing	Acidifying	Strongly Acidifying	Moderate Salicylates	Very High Salicylates	Sulfites	Amines	High Amines	MSG	High Glycemic Index	Gluten	Additives	Severe Reactions
Pumpernickel			•									•		
Quinoa, red or white			•								•			
Rice crackers, plain				•							•			
Rice milk			•											
Rye flour			•									•		
Soy flour			•											
Spelt pasta			•									•		
Spelt bread			•									•		
Sweet potato		•			•									
Tapioca (sago)			•								•			
White bread				•							•	•		
Sprouted grains		•										•		
Wheat cereals				•							•	•		
White rice, jasmine				•							•			
Whole-grain wheat bread			•									•		
Yeast breads			•									•		
PROTEIN: MEAT, DAIRY, LEGUMES														
Anchovies			•						•					
Beans (not fava)			•											
Beans, fava			•		•									
Beef				•										
Butter, heated				•										
Butter, pure, unheated		•												
Buttermilk, fresh		•												
Cheese				•					•					
Chicken			•											
Chickpeas (garbanzo beans)			•											
Deli meats				•		•			•	•			•	•
Egg			•											•
Fish, fresh			•				•							
Fish, pickled, smoked				•					•					

	Strongly Alkalizing	Alkalizing	Acidifying	Strongly Acidifying	Moderate Salicylates	Very High Salicylates	Sulfites	Amines	High Amines	MSG	High Glycemic Index	Gluten	Additives	Severe Reactions
Ghee (clarified butter)		•												
Ice cream			•								•		•	
Kefir			•											
Lamb, lean			•											
Lentils			•											
Lobster			•											
Meat pies			•						•	•			•	
Milk, dairy			•											•
Milk, soy, organic			•									•		
Peanut			•		•				•					
Pork, ham, bacon			•						•	•			•	
Salmon			•					•						
Sausages			•		•			•		•			•	
Tempeh		•							•	•				
Tuna, canned in olive oil		•			•				•					
Tuna, canned in springwater		•							•					
Veal		•												
Whey, fresh		•												
Yogurt, plain, organic		•												
Yogurt, sweetened, fruit			•		•									
NUTS AND SEEDS														
Almonds		•			•				•					
Almond milk		•			•				•					
Brazil nuts		•			•									
Cashews, raw, unsalted		•												
Cashews, roasted			•		•				•					
Coconut			•		•				•					
Hazelnuts				•	•				•					
Pine nuts			•		•				•					
Pistachio nuts				•	•				•					
Pumpkin seeds				•	•				•					

	Strongly Alkalizing	Alkalizing	Acidifying	Strongly Acidifying	Moderate Salicylates	Very High Salicylates	Sulfites	Amines	High Amines	MSG	High Glycemic Index	Gluten	Additives	Severe Reactions
Sesame seeds			•		•				•					
Sunflower seeds			•		•				•					
Walnuts				•	•				•					
FATS AND OILS														
Almond oil		•		•										
Butter, pure		•												
Canola oil			•										•	
Flaxseed oil		•		•										
Hydrogenated fats				•										
Lard				•										
Olive oil, extra virgin		•			•				•					
Rice bran oil			•											
Safflower oil			•											
Margarine				•									•	•
CONDIMENTS, SWEETENERS AND FLAVORINGS														
Apple cider vinegar	•				•	•			•					•
Artificial sweeteners				•									•	•
Barley malt			•									•		
Carob powder			•											
Celtic sea salt, unrefined		•												
Chewing gum and candy				•		•							•	•
Chives		•												
Chocolate				•					•				•	
Curry powder and paste		•			•									•
Cinnamon		•			•									
Garlic		•												
Ginger		•			•									
Golden syrup				•										
Gravy				•		•	•		•	•				

	Strongly Alkalizing	Alkalizing	Acidifying	Strongly Acidifying	Moderate Salicylates	Very High Salicylates	Sulfites	Amines	High Amines	MSG	High Glycemic Index	Gluten	Additives	Severe Reactions
Herbs		•				•								
Honey			•			•								
Hydrolyzed vegetable protein			•						•	•				
Jams			•			•	•							
Lecithin granules, soy		•												
Licorice			•			•								
Mayonnaise				•		•			•				•	•
Maple syrup, pure			•											
Meat extracts				•		•				•				
Molasses			•		•									
Mustard				•		•			•					•
Rice malt syrup		•												
Saffron		•												
Salt, table				•									•	
Spices		•				•								
Soy sauce			•						•	•		•	•	
Stock cubes			•			•			•	•			•	
Tomato sauces				•		•		•	•				•	
Vanilla, extract			•											
Vanilla, whole bean		•												
Vinegars				•	•	•	•							
BEVERAGES, BROTHS, SOUPS														
Beer			•		•		•	•						
Black tea				•		•	•							
Broth, homemade	•													
Chocolate drinks				•					•				•	
Coffee				•	•								•	
Cordial				•		•							•	
Fruit juice			•			•	•							
Green detox powder	•					•								•
Green tea			•			•								

	Strongly Alkalizing	Alkalizing	Acidifying	Strongly Acidifying	Moderate Salicylates	Very High Salicylates	Sulfites	Amines	High Amines	MSG	High Glycemic Index	Gluten	Additives	Severe Reactions
Healthy Skin Juice	•				•									
Herbal teas (not green tea)		•			•									
Tarzan Juice	•													
Liquor, brandy, whiskey, rum			•		•				•					
Liquid chlorophyll	•				•									
Milk, dairy			•											•
Mineral water, carbonated			•											
Mineral water, not carbonated		•												
Rice milk, plain, organic			•								•			
Soft drinks, soda, pop				•	•						•		•	
Soup mixes, dried				•	•	•				•	•	•	•	
Soy milk, plain, organic			•								•			
Soy milk, organic, malt free			•											
Tomato juice and soup			•			•	•	•		•				
Vegetable juice, packaged			•			•	•	•		•				
Vegetable juice, raw	•				•									
Water, filtered		•												
Water, tap				•										
Wine				•		•	•		•	•			•	•

Chapter 10
Menu Plans

• •

Menu planning is one cornerstone of the Eczema Diet. At the beginning, follow the plans quite closely. Once you get the hang of it, introduce new meals from the recipe section.

Five Goals of Menu Planning

1. Eat 5 or more servings of eczema-safe vegetables per day to reap the benefits of their antioxidant and alkalizing properties. This is an important step in preventing eczema — and in preventing its recurrence.

2. You need to consume 2 servings of fruit to meet your daily vitamin C and potassium requirements. Do not eat too much fruit, especially if you have any signs of fungal overgrowth, dandruff, or *Candida albicans*. If you are craving sweets, another piece of fruit is allowed.

3. You must eat at least 2 servings of whole grains daily to ensure you are consuming sufficient dietary fiber to promote healthy microflora and to cleanse the bowel of toxins and carcinogens.

4. You must eat two protein ingredients daily to ensure you are consuming enough protein for skin repair and maintenance. Protein-rich foods are usually good sources of iron, which is vital for healthy skin. If you are vegan, you may require an iron supplement.

5. Drink 5 to 8 glasses, or 48 to 64 ounces (1.5 to 2 L), of liquids to hydrate the gastrointestinal tract and your skin. Each glass of filtered water, eczema-safe vegetable juice (such as Tarzan Juice, page 207), organic rice milk, Therapeutic Broth (page 212), or soup counts for liquid intake.

Children's Menu Plan

	Monday (day 1)	Tuesday (2)	Wednesday (3)
Breakfast	Supplements with Tarzan Juice, p. 207, filtered water or rice milk ***Choose from:*** Surprise Porridge, p. 199; Omega Muesli, p. 198; plain rice cereal with rice milk; or Quinoa Porridge, p. 200	Supplements with Tarzan Juice, p. 207, filtered water or rice milk ***Choose from:*** Surprise Porridge, p. 199; plain rice cereal with rice milk; Quinoa Porridge, p. 200; or Omega Muesli, p. 198	Supplements with Tarzan Juice, p. 207, filtered water or rice milk ***Choose from:*** Surprise Porridge, p. 199; plain rice cereal with rice milk; Quinoa Porridge, p. 200; or Omega Muesli, p. 198 with Baked Banana Chips, p. 242 (or banana)
Morning Snack *("Morning tea is fruit time")*	***Choose from:*** papaya, banana and/or pear; plain rice crackers; Pear Muffin, p. 203; Baked Banana Chips, p. 242; spelt mini pancakes with rice malt syrup and banana (use Spelt Pancake recipe, p. 201); or Healthy Skin Smoothie, p. 209 Filtered water	***Choose from:*** papaya balls (use a melon baller), banana and/or pear; plain rice crackers; Pear Muffin, p. 203; Baked Banana Chips, p. 242; spelt mini pancakes with rice malt syrup and banana (use Spelt Pancake recipe, p. 201); or Healthy Skin Smoothie, p. 209 Filtered water	***Choose from:*** papaya, banana and/or pear; plain rice crackers; Pear Muffin, p. 203; Baked Banana Chips, p. 242; spelt mini pancakes with rice malt syrup and banana (use Spelt Pancake recipe, p. 201) or Healthy Skin Smoothie, p. 209 Filtered water
Lunch *("Brainy grain time")*	***Choose from:*** Design Your Own Sandwich, p. 223; or Pasta with beans, chicken or fish, p. 230 Filtered water	***Choose from:*** Design Your Own Sandwich, p. 223; or Pasta with beans, chicken or fish, p. 230 Filtered water	***Choose from:*** Design Your Own Sandwich, p. 223; or Pasta with beans, chicken or fish, p. 230 Filtered water
Afternoon Snack *("Afternoon tea is veggie time")*	***Choose from:*** carrot and celery sticks, rice crackers and Sesame-Free Hummus, p. 239 or Bean Dip, p. 240; Wishing Plate, p. 245; or Alkaline Bomb Salad, p. 218 Tarzan Juice, p. 207, Healthy Skin Juice, p. 206 or filtered water	***Choose from:*** carrot and celery sticks, rice crackers and Sesame-Free Hummus, p. 239 or Bean Dip, p. 240; or Alkaline Bomb Salad, p. 218 Tarzan Juice, p. 207 or filtered water	***Choose from:*** carrot and celery sticks, rice crackers and Sesame-Free Hummus, p. 239 or Bean Dip, p. 240; Wishing Plate p. 245; or Alkaline Bomb Salad, p. 218 Tarzan Juice, p. 207 or filtered water
Dinner	***Choose from:*** Chickpea Casserole, p. 224, or soup of choice, pp. 215–217 ***Optional Dessert:*** frozen banana slices, eczema-safe fruits, or Pear Muffin, p. 203 Filtered water or rice milk	***Choose from:*** New Potato and Leek Soup, p. 215 with gluten-free bread or Spelt Lavash Bread, p. 243, or use up leftovers Filtered water or rice milk	***Choose from:*** Cinnamon Chicken, p. 227 (don't use cinnamon); or use up leftover soup Filtered water or rice milk
Rate your child's eczema:	___/10	___/10	___/10

Thursday (4)	Friday (5)	Saturday (6)	Sunday (7 - *treat day*)
Supplements with Tarzan Juice, p. 207, filtered water or rice milk *Choose from:* Surprise Porridge, p. 199; plain rice cereal with rice milk; Quinoa Porridge, p. 200; or Omega Muesli, p. 198	Supplements with Tarzan Juice, p. 207, filtered water or rice milk *Choose from:* Surprise Porridge, p. 199; plain rice cereal with rice milk; Quinoa Porridge, p. 200; or Omega Muesli, p. 198	Supplements with Tarzan Juice, p. 207, filtered water or rice milk *Choose from:* Surprise Porridge, p. 199; plain rice cereal with rice milk; Quinoa Porridge, p. 200; or Omega Muesli, p. 198	Supplements with Tarzan Juice, p. 207, filtered water or rice milk *Choose from:* Spelt Pancakes, p. 201; plain rice cereal with rice milk; Buckwheat Crêpes, p. 202; or Healthy Skin Smoothie, p. 209
Choose from: papaya, banana and/or pear; plain rice crackers; Pear Muffin, p. 203; Baked Banana Chips, p. 242; spelt mini pancakes with rice malt syrup and banana (use Spelt Pancake recipe, p. 201); or Healthy Skin Smoothie, p. 209 Filtered water	*Choose from:* papaya, banana and/or pear; plain rice crackers; Pear Muffin, p. 203; Baked Banana Chips, p. 242; spelt mini pancakes with rice malt syrup and banana (use Spelt Pancake recipe, p. 201); or Healthy Skin Smoothie, p. 209 Filtered water	*Choose from:* papaya, banana and/or pear; plain rice crackers; Pear Muffin, p. 203; Baked Banana Chips, p. 242; spelt mini pancakes with rice malt syrup and banana (use Spelt Pancake recipe, p. 201) or Healthy Skin Smoothie, p. 209 Filtered water	*Choose from:* papaya, banana and/or pear; Pear Muffin, p. 203; spelt mini pancakes with rice malt syrup and banana (use Spelt Pancake recipe, p. 201); vanilla soy yogurt (no E160b/annatto) with fresh pear; or Healthy Skin Smoothie, p. 209 Filtered water
Choose from: Design Your Own Sandwich, p. 223 Filtered water	*Choose from:* Design Your Own Sandwich, p. 223; or Pasta with beans, chicken or fish, p. 230 Filtered water	*Choose from:* Design Your Own Sandwich, p. 223; or Pasta with beans, chicken or fish, p. 230 Filtered water	*Choose from:* Design Your Own Sandwich, p. 223; or Pasta with beans, chicken or fish, p. 230 Filtered water
Choose from: carrot and celery sticks, rice crackers and Sesame-Free Hummus, p. 239 or Bean Dip, p. 240; Wishing Plate p. 245; or Alkaline Bomb Salad, p. 218 Tarzan Juice, p. 207, Healthy Skin Juice, p. 206 or filtered water	*Choose from:* carrot and celery sticks, rice crackers and Sesame-Free Hummus, p. 239 or Bean Dip, p. 240; Wishing Plate p. 245; or Alkaline Bomb Salad, p. 218 Tarzan Juice, p. 207, or filtered water	*Choose from:* carrot and celery sticks, rice crackers and Sesame-Free Hummus, p. 239 or Bean Dip, p. 240; Wishing Plate, p. 245; or Alkaline Bomb Salad, p. 218 Tarzan Juice, p. 207 or filtered water	*Choose from:* carrot and celery sticks, rice crackers and Sesame-Free Hummus, p. 239 or Bean Dip, p. 240; Wishing Plate p. 245; or Alkaline Bomb Salad, p. 218 Tarzan Juice, p. 207, Healthy Skin Juice, p. 206 or filtered water
Choose from: Baked Fish with Mash, p. 225 or use up leftovers; or soup of choice, pp. 215–217 Filtered water or rice milk	*Choose from:* Country Chicken Soup, p. 217, or Papaya Rice Paper Rolls, p. 222; or soup of choice, pp. 215–217 *Optional Dessert:* frozen banana slices Filtered water or rice milk	*Choose from:* Sticks and Stones, p. 226 or use up leftovers; or soup of choice, pp. 215–217 Filtered water or rice milk	*Choose from:* Easy Roast Chicken, p. 228 or soup of choice, pp. 215–217 *Optional Dessert:* Banana on Sticks, p. 252; Banana Icy Pole, p. 251; or Spelt Pancakes, p. 201 Filtered water, rice milk or Chocolate Milk, p. 210
___/10	___/10	___/10	___/10

	Monday (day 8)	Tuesday (9)	Wednesday (10)
Breakfast	Supplements with Tarzan Juice, p. 207, filtered water or rice milk *Choose from:* Surprise Porridge, p. 199; plain rice cereal with rice milk; Quinoa Porridge, p. 200; or Omega Muesli, p. 198 with Baked Banana Chips, p. 242 (or banana)	Supplements with Tarzan Juice, p. 207, filtered water or rice milk *Choose from:* Surprise Porridge, p. 199; plain rice cereal with rice milk; Quinoa Porridge, p. 200; Omega Muesli, p. 198 with Baked Banana Chips, p. 242 (or banana)	Supplements with Tarzan Juice, p. 207, filtered water or rice milk *Choose from:* Surprise Porridge, p. 199; plain rice cereal with rice milk; Quinoa Porridge, p. 200; Omega Muesli, p. 198 with Baked Banana Chips, p. 242 (or banana)
Morning Snack ("*Morning tea is fruit time*")	*Choose from:* papaya, banana and/or pear; multigrain rye crackers; Pear Muffin, p. 203; Baked Banana Chips, p. 242; spelt mini pancakes with rice malt syrup and banana (use Spelt Pancake recipe, p. 201); or Healthy Skin Smoothie, p. 209 Filtered water	*Choose from:* papaya, banana and/or pear; multigrain rye crackers; Pear Muffin, p. 203; Baked Banana Chips, p. 242; spelt mini pancakes with rice malt syrup and banana (use Spelt Pancake recipe, p. 201); or Healthy Skin Smoothie, p. 209 Filtered water	*Choose from:* papaya, banana and/or pear; multigrain rye crackers; Pear Muffin, p. 203; Baked Banana Chips, p. 242; spelt mini pancakes with rice malt syrup and banana (use Spelt Pancake recipe, p. 201); or Healthy Skin Smoothie, p. 209 Filtered water
Lunch ("*Brainy grain time*")	*Choose from:* Design Your Own Sandwich, p. 223; or Pasta with beans, chicken or fish, p. 230 Filtered water	*Choose from:* Design Your Own Sandwich, p. 223; or Pasta with beans, chicken or fish, p. 230 Filtered water	*Choose from:* Design Your Own Sandwich, p. 223; or Pasta with beans, chicken or fish, p. 230 Filtered water
Afternoon Snack ("*Afternoon tea is veggie time*")	*Choose from:* carrot and celery sticks, rice crackers and Sesame-Free Hummus, p. 239 or Bean Dip, p. 240; Wishing Plate p. 245; or Alkaline Bomb Salad, p. 218 Tarzan Juice, p. 207, or filtered water	*Choose from:* carrot and celery sticks, rice crackers and Sesame-Free Hummus, p. 239 or Bean Dip, p. 240; Wishing Plate p. 245; or Alkaline Bomb Salad, p. 218 Tarzan Juice, p. 207 or filtered water	*Choose from:* carrot and celery sticks, rice crackers and Sesame-Free Hummus, p. 239 or Bean Dip, p. 240; Wishing Plate p. 245; or Alkaline Bomb Salad, p. 218 Tarzan Juice, p. 207, Healthy Skin Juice, p. 206 or filtered water
Dinner	*Choose from:* Chickpea Rice, p. 234 (with leftover chicken) or use up leftovers; or soup of choice, pp. 215–217 Filtered water or rice milk	*Choose from:* Sunshine Soup, p. 216; or My Favorite Lamb Chops, p. 231; or use up leftovers; or soup of choice, pp. 215–217 *Dessert:* papaya (rich in vitamin C to help iron absorption) Filtered water or rice milk	*Choose from:* Chickpea Casserole, p. 224 or Papaya Rice Paper Rolls, p. 222; or soup of choice, pp. 215–217 Filtered water or rice milk
Rate your child's eczema:	___/10	___/10	___/10

Thursday (11)	Friday (12)	Saturday (13)	Sunday (14 - *treat day*)
Supplements with Tarzan Juice, p. 207, filtered water or rice milk *Choose from:* Surprise Porridge, p. 199; plain rice cereal with rice milk; Quinoa Porridge, p. 200; Omega Muesli, p. 198 with Baked Banana Chips, p. 242 (or banana)	Supplements with Tarzan Juice, p. 207, filtered water or rice milk *Choose from:* Surprise Porridge, p. 199; plain rice cereal with rice milk; Quinoa Porridge, p. 200; Omega Muesli, p. 198 with Baked Banana Chips, p. 242 (or banana)	Supplements with Tarzan Juice, p. 207, filtered water or rice milk *Choose from:* Surprise Porridge, p. 199; plain rice cereal with rice milk; Quinoa Porridge, p. 200; Omega Muesli, p. 198 with Baked Banana Chips, p. 242 (or banana)	Supplements with Tarzan Juice, p. 207, filtered water or rice milk *Choose from:* Spelt Pancakes, p. 201; plain rice cereal with rice milk; Buckwheat Crêpes, p. 202 (GF option) or Healthy Skin Smoothie, p. 209
Choose from: papaya, banana and/or pear; multigrain rye crackers; Pear Muffin, p. 203; Baked Banana Chips, p. 242; spelt mini pancakes with rice malt syrup and banana (use Spelt Pancake recipe, p. 201); or Healthy Skin Smoothie, p. 209 Filtered water	*Choose from:* papaya, banana and/or pear; multigrain rye crackers; Pear Muffin, p. 203; Baked Banana Chips, p. 242; spelt mini pancakes with rice malt syrup and banana (use Spelt Pancake recipe, p. 201); or Healthy Skin Smoothie, p. 209 Filtered water	*Choose from:* papaya, banana and/or pear; multigrain rye crackers; Pear Muffin, p. 203; Baked Banana Chips, p. 242; spelt mini pancakes with rice malt syrup and banana (use Spelt Pancake recipe, p. 201); or Healthy Skin Smoothie, p. 209 Filtered water	*Choose from:* papaya balls (using a melon baller), banana and/or pear; Pear Muffin, p. 203; spelt mini pancakes with rice malt syrup and banana (use Spelt Pancake recipe, p. 201); vanilla soy yogurt (no E160b/annatto) with fresh pear; or Healthy Skin Smoothie, p. 209 Filtered water
Choose from: Design Your Own Sandwich, p. 223; or Pasta with beans, chicken or fish, p. 230 Filtered water	*Choose from:* Design Your Own Sandwich, p. 223; or Pasta with beans, chicken or fish, p. 230 Filtered water	*Choose from:* Design Your Own Sandwich, p. 223; or Pasta with beans, chicken or fish, p. 230 Filtered water	*Choose from:* Design Your Own Sandwich, p. 223; or Pasta with beans, chicken or fish, p. 230 Filtered water
Choose from: carrot and celery sticks, rice crackers and Sesame-Free Hummus, p. 239 or Bean Dip, p. 240; Wishing Plate p. 245; or Alkaline Bomb Salad, p. 218 Tarzan Juice, p. 207, Healthy Skin Juice, p. 206 or filtered water	*Choose from:* carrot and celery sticks, rice crackers and Sesame-Free Hummus, p. 239 or Bean Dip, p. 240; Wishing Plate p. 245; or Alkaline Bomb Salad, p. 218 Tarzan Juice, p. 207, Healthy Skin Juice, p. 206 or filtered water	*Choose from:* carrot and celery sticks, rice crackers and Sesame-Free Hummus, p. 239 or Bean Dip, p. 240; Wishing Plate p. 245; or Alkaline Bomb Salad, p. 218 Tarzan Juice, p. 207, or filtered water	*Choose from:* carrot and celery sticks, rice crackers and Sesame-Free Hummus, p. 239 or Bean Dip, p. 240; Wishing Plate p. 245; or Alkaline Bomb Salad, p. 218 Tarzan Juice, p. 207, Healthy Skin Juice, p. 206 or filtered water
Choose from: Chicken Pasta with Green Beans, p. 230 or use up leftovers; or soup of choice, pp. 215–217 Filtered water or rice milk	*Choose from:* My Favorite Lamb Chops, p. 231; or use up leftovers; or soup of choice, pp. 215–217 *Dessert:* papaya (rich in vitamin C to help iron absorption) Filtered water or rice milk	*Choose from:* Baked Fish with Mash, p. 225 (use catfish or eczema-safe white fish, p. 69); or soup of choice, pp. 215–217 Filtered water or rice milk	*Choose from:* Easy Roast Chicken, p. 228 (or use a lean cut of lamb); or soup of choice, pp. 215–217 *Optional Dessert:* Banana on Sticks, p. 252, Banana Icy Pole, p. 251, or Spelt Pancakes, p. 201 Filtered water, rice milk or Chocolate Milk, p. 210
___/10	___/10	___/10	___/10

Lunch Box Menu: A (ages 1–3 years)

	Monday (day 1)	Tuesday (2)
Mid-Morning Snack	Choose from: peeled pear; papaya; banana (not sugar variety), and/or Pear Muffin, p. 203 Water bottle (filtered water)	Choose from: papaya balls (use a melon baller); banana Water bottle (filtered water)
Lunch	Design Your Own Sandwich, p. 223 or *gluten-free pasta spirals with lamb, kidney beans and soft carrot or green beans Pack a spoon and freezer block	Design Your Own Sandwich, p. 223 or wheat-free sandwich with diced/sliced chicken (home-cooked or organic) with grated carrot or shredded iceberg lettuce, pack a freezer block
Afternoon Snack	Celery cut into "shark's teeth" shapes (not sticks as they may be too chewy) and plain rice crackers or Spelt Chips (variation, p. 243)	Spelt Chips (variation, p. 243) and serve with Sesame-Free Hummus, p. 239

Lunch Box Menu: B (age 3+ years)

	Monday (day 1)	Tuesday (2)
Mid-Morning Snack	Choose from: peeled and sliced pear; papaya; plain rice cakes/crackers; and Baked Banana Chips, p. 242 Water bottle (filtered water)	Choose from: papaya balls (use a melon baller); banana (not sugar variety); plain rice cakes/crackers Water bottle (filtered water)
Lunch	Design Your Own Sandwich, p. 223 or *gluten-free pasta spirals with lamb, kidney beans and soft carrot or green beans Pack a spoon and freezer block	Design Your Own Sandwich, p. 223 or wheat-free sandwich with thinly sliced chicken (home-cooked or organic) with shredded iceberg lettuce Pack a spoon and freezer block
Afternoon Snack	Carrot sticks with Sesame-Free Hummus, p. 239 or Bean Dip, p. 240, and Spelt Chips (variation, p. 243)	Peeled celery sticks with Sesame-Free Hummus, p. 239 (spread in groove), and Spelt Chips (variation, p. 243).

Wednesday (3)	Thursday (4)	Friday (5 - treat day)
Pear Muffin, p. 203; banana Water bottle (filtered water)	Choose from: peeled pear and papaya balls; plain rice cakes/crackers Water bottle (filtered water)	Choose from: banana; peeled pear slices and celery cut into "shark's teeth" shapes (not sticks as they may be too chewy) Water bottle (filtered water)
Design Your Own Sandwich, p. 223 or wheat-free sandwich with Banana Carob Spread, p. 238	Design Your Own Sandwich, p. 223 or *"Potato Man" (kidney/green beans, carrot and/or celery slotted into a baked potato to make a "potato man" — serve with extra kidney beans in an iceberg lettuce leaf "cup") Pack a spoon and freezer block	Design Your Own Sandwich, p. 223 or wheat-free sandwich with Banana Carob Spread, p. 238
"Shark's teeth" celery slices, and vanilla soy yogurt (no E160b or "natural color" annatto) with chopped canned pear and papaya Pack a spoon and freezer block	Spelt Chips (variation, p. 243) and serve with Bean Dip, p. 240	New Anzac Cookies, p. 250 and/or vanilla soy yogurt (no E160b or "natural color" annatto) topped with Banana Carob Spread, p. 238; or papaya and chopped canned pear Pack a spoon and freezer block

*(*You can use dinner leftovers for lunch, and most of the recipes in Chapter 18 are suitable. Just be sure to adjust the portions and cut up foods into smaller bite-sizes to suit your child's age and feeding ability.)*

Wednesday (3)	Thursday (4)	Friday (5 - treat day)
Pear Muffin, p. 203 and a banana Water bottle (filtered water) Pack a freezer block	Choose from: papaya; peeled pear (pack a fork); plain rice cakes/crackers Water bottle (filtered water)	Choose from: Pear Muffin, p. 203; banana; or Papaya Rice Paper Rolls, p. 222 Water bottle (filtered water)
Design Your Own Sandwich, p. 223 or Papaya Rice Paper Rolls, p. 222	Design Your Own Sandwich, p. 223 or *potato salad with diced potato, kidney beans, celery and iceberg lettuce (and diced papaya for sweetness) Pack a spoon and freezer block	Design Your Own Sandwich, p. 223 or wheat-free sandwich with Banana Carob Spread, p. 238
Plain rice crackers and peeled carrot sticks with Bean Dip, p. 240	Spelt Chips (variation, p. 243) and serve with Sesame-Free Hummus, p. 239 or Parsley Pesto, p. 241 (contains cashews so may not be allowed at school)	New Anzac Cookies, p. 250 or vanilla soy yogurt (no E160b or "natural color" annatto) with Banana Carob Spread, p. 238 or papaya and chopped canned pear Pack a spoon and freezer block

*(*You can use dinner leftovers for lunch, and most of the recipes in Chapter 18 are suitable. Just be sure to adjust the portions and cut up foods into smaller bite-sizes to suit your child's age and feeding ability.)*

Adult/Family Menu Plan

	Monday (day 1)	Tuesday (2)	Wednesday (3)
Breakfast	Supplements with filtered water or Tarzan Juice, p. 207 Baked potatoes (no oil) with celery and mung bean sprouts; optional: ½ cup warm broth	Supplements with filtered water or Tarzan Juice, p. 207 *Choose from:* baked potato (no oil) with celery and mung bean sprouts; or New Potato and Leek Soup, p. 215	Supplements with filtered water or Tarzan Juice, p. 207 *Choose from:* baked potato (no oil) with celery and mung bean sprouts; or New Potato and Leek Soup, p. 215
Morning Snack	*Choose from:* salad: iceberg lettuce, celery, mung bean sprouts, spring onion (scallions); or steamed baby potatoes and green beans topped with chopped chives Tarzan Juice, p. 207 or filtered water	*Choose from:* salad: iceberg lettuce, celery, mung bean sprouts, spring onion (scallions); or steamed baby potatoes and green beans topped with chopped chives Tarzan Juice, p. 207 or filtered water	*Choose from:* salad: iceberg lettuce, celery, mung bean sprouts, spring onion (scallions); or steamed baby potatoes and green beans topped with chopped chives Tarzan Juice, p. 207 or filtered water
Lunch	New Potato and Leek Soup, p. 215 Filtered water	New Potato and Leek Soup, p. 215 Filtered water	New Potato and Leek Soup, p. 215 Filtered water
Afternoon Snack	*Choose from:* salad: iceberg lettuce, celery, mung bean sprouts, spring onion (scallions); or steamed baby potatoes and green beans topped with chopped chives Tarzan Juice, p. 207 or filtered water	*Choose from:* salad: iceberg lettuce, celery, mung bean sprouts, spring onion (scallions); or steamed baby potatoes and green beans topped with chopped chives Tarzan Juice, p. 207 or filtered water	*Choose from:* salad: iceberg lettuce, celery, mung bean sprouts, spring onion (scallions); or steamed baby potatoes and green beans topped with chopped chives Tarzan Juice, p. 207 or filtered water
Dinner	Chickpea Casserole, p. 224 (1–2 serves, do not go hungry) Filtered water	Chickpea Casserole, p. 224 (1–2 serves, do not go hungry) Filtered water	Chickpea Casserole, p. 224 (1–2 serves, do not go hungry) Filtered water (Soak oats or quinoa for tomorrow's breakfast, see day 4, opposite)
Rate your eczema:	___/10	___/10	___/10

Thursday (4)	Friday (5)	Saturday (6)	Sunday (7 - *treat day*)
Supplements with filtered water or Healthy Skin Juice, p. 206 *Choose from:* Omega Muesli, p. 198; Surprise Porridge, p. 199; Quinoa Porridge, p. 200; or Healthy Skin Smoothie, p. 209 (Make Therapeutic Broth if you have run out, p. 212)	Supplements with filtered water or Tarzan Juice, p. 207 *Choose from:* Omega Muesli, p. 198; Surprise Porridge, p. 199; Quinoa Porridge, p. 200; or Healthy Skin Smoothie, p. 209	Supplements with filtered water or Healthy Skin Juice, p. 206 *Choose from:* Omega Muesli, p. 198; Surprise Porridge, p. 199; Quinoa Porridge, p. 200; or Healthy Skin Smoothie, p. 209	Supplements with filtered water or Tarzan Juice, p. 207 *Choose from:* Omega Muesli, p. 198; Spelt Pancakes, p. 201; Buckwheat Crêpes, p. 202; or Healthy Skin Smoothie, p. 209
Choose from: papaya, banana or peeled pear; Eczema-Safe Fruit Salad, p. 246; or Healthy Skin Smoothie, p. 209 Filtered water and/or Healthy Skin Juice, p. 206	*Choose from:* papaya, banana or peeled pear; Eczema-Safe Fruit Salad, p. 246; or Healthy Skin Smoothie, p. 209 Filtered water and/or Healthy Skin Juice, p. 206	*Choose from:* papaya, banana or peeled pear; Eczema-Safe Fruit Salad, p. 246; or Healthy Skin Smoothie, p. 209 Filtered water and/or Healthy Skin Juice, p. 206	*Choose from:* Banana Icy Pole, p. 251, papaya or peeled pear; Eczema-Safe Fruit Salad, p. 246; or Healthy Skin Smoothie, p. 209 Filtered water and/or Healthy Skin Juice, p. 206
Choose from: Design Your Own Sandwich, p. 223; Papaya Rice Paper Rolls, p. 222; Roasted Sweet Potato Salad, p. 219; or Roasted Potato Snack, p. 244 (all have GF options) Filtered water	*Choose from:* Design Your Own Sandwich, p. 223; Papaya Rice Paper Rolls, p. 222; Roasted Sweet Potato Salad, p. 219; or Roasted Potato Snack, p. 244 (all have GF options) Filtered water	*Choose from:* Design Your Own Sandwich, p. 223; Papaya Rice Paper Rolls, p. 222; Roasted Sweet Potato Salad, p. 219; or Roasted Potato Snack, p. 244 (all have GF options) Filtered water	*Choose from:* Spelt Lavash Bread, p. 243 with salad or Banana Carob Spread, p. 238; Design Your Own Sandwich, p. 223; Papaya Rice Paper Rolls, p. 222; or Roasted Potato Snack, p. 244 (all have GF options) Filtered water
Choose from: carrot and celery sticks with Sesame-Free Hummus, p. 239 and brown rice crackers; or Alkaline Bomb Salad, p. 218 Filtered water or Healthy Skin Juice, p. 206	*Choose from:* carrot and celery sticks with Sesame-Free Hummus, p. 239 and brown rice crackers; or Alkaline Bomb Salad, p. 218 Filtered water or Tarzan Juice, p. 207	*Choose from:* carrot and celery sticks with Sesame-Free Hummus, p. 239 and brown rice crackers; or Alkaline Bomb Salad, p. 218 Filtered water or Healthy Skin Juice, p. 206	*Choose from:* carrot and celery sticks with Sesame-Free Hummus, p. 239 and brown rice crackers; Alkaline Bomb Salad, p. 218; or Potato Wedges, p. 233 and Sesame-Free Hummus, p. 239 Filtered water or Tarzan Juice, p. 207
Choose from: Baked Fish with Mash, p. 225; or soup of choice, pp. 215–217	*Choose from:* Cinnamon Chicken, p. 227; or soup of choice, pp. 215–217	*Choose from:* Sticks and Stones, p. 226 (skewers); or soup of choice, pp. 215–217	*Choose from:* Easy Roast Chicken, p. 228; or soup of choice, pp. 215–217 Chickpea Rice, p. 234 (V&Vn) *Optional Dessert:* Chocolate Milk, p. 210; Banana Icy Poles, p. 251; or Baked Banana Chips, p. 242
___/10	___/10	___/10	___/10

	Monday (day 8)	Tuesday (9)	Wednesday (10)
Breakfast	Supplements with filtered water or Healthy Skin Juice, p. 206 *Choose from:* Omega Muesli, p. 198; Surprise Porridge, p. 199; Quinoa Porridge, p. 200; or Healthy Skin Smoothie, p. 209 (Make Therapeutic Broth if you have run out, p. 212)	Supplements with filtered water or Tarzan Juice, p. 207 *Choose from:* Omega Muesli, p. 198; Surprise Porridge, p. 199; Quinoa Porridge, p. 200; or Healthy Skin Smoothie, p. 209	Supplements with filtered water or Healthy Skin Juice, p. 206 *Choose from:* Omega Muesli, p. 198; Surprise Porridge, p. 199; Quinoa Porridge, p. 200; or Healthy Skin Smoothie, p. 209
Morning Snack	*Choose from:* papaya, banana or peeled pear; Eczema-Safe Fruit Salad, p. 246; or Healthy Skin Smoothie, p. 209 Filtered water and/or Healthy Skin Juice, p. 206	*Choose from:* papaya, banana or peeled pear; Eczema-Safe Fruit Salad, p. 246; or Healthy Skin Smoothie, p. 209 Filtered water and/or Healthy Skin Juice, p. 206	*Choose from:* papaya, banana or peeled pear; Eczema-Safe Fruit Salad, p. 246; or Healthy Skin Smoothie, p. 209 Filtered water and/or Healthy Skin Juice, p. 206
Lunch	*Choose from:* Design Your Own Sandwich, p. 223; Papaya Rice Paper Rolls, p. 222; Roasted Sweet Potato Salad, p. 219; or Roasted Potato Snack, p. 244 (all have GF options) Filtered water	*Choose from:* Design Your Own Sandwich, p. 223; Papaya Rice Paper Rolls, p. 222; Roasted Sweet Potato Salad, p. 219; or Roasted Potato Snack, p. 244 (all have GF options) Filtered water	*Choose from:* Design Your Own Sandwich, p. 223; Papaya Rice Paper Rolls, p. 222; Roasted Sweet Potato Salad, p. 219; or Roasted Potato Snack, p. 244 (all have GF options) Filtered water
Afternoon Snack	*Choose from:* carrot and celery sticks with Sesame-Free Hummus, p. 239 and brown rice crackers; or Alkaline Bomb Salad, p. 218 Filtered water or Healthy Skin Juice, p. 206	*Choose from:* carrot and celery sticks with Sesame-Free Hummus, p. 239 and brown rice crackers; or Alkaline Bomb Salad, p. 218 Filtered water or Tarzan Juice, p. 207	*Choose from:* carrot and celery sticks with Sesame-Free Hummus, p. 239 and brown rice crackers; or Alkaline Bomb Salad, p. 218 Filtered water or Healthy Skin Juice, p. 206
Dinner	*Choose from:* Chickpea Rice, p. 234 (with leftover roast chicken); or soup of choice, pp. 215–217	*Choose from:* Sunshine Soup, p. 216; or soup of choice, pp. 215–217	*Choose from:* Chickpea Casserole, p. 224; Papaya Rice Paper Rolls, p. 222 (served with rice or salad); or soup of choice, pp. 215–217
Rate your eczema:	___/10	___/10	___/10

Thursday (11)	Friday (12)	Saturday (13)	Sunday (14 - *treat day*)
Supplements with filtered water or Tarzan Juice, p. 207 *Choose from:* Omega Muesli, p. 198; Surprise Porridge, p. 199; Quinoa Porridge, p. 200; or Healthy Skin Smoothie, p. 209	Supplements with filtered water or Healthy Skin Juice, p. 206 *Choose from:* Omega Muesli, p. 198; Surprise Porridge, p. 199; Quinoa Porridge, p. 200; or Healthy Skin Smoothie, p. 209 (Make Therapeutic Broth if you have run out, p. 212)	Supplements with filtered water or Tarzan Juice, p. 207 *Choose from:* Omega Muesli, p. 198; Surprise Porridge, p. 199; Quinoa Porridge, p. 200; or Healthy Skin Smoothie, p. 209	Supplements with filtered water or Healthy Skin Juice, p. 206 *Choose from:* Omega Muesli, p. 198; Spelt Pancakes, p. 201; Buckwheat Crêpes, p. 202; or Healthy Skin Smoothie, p. 209
Choose from: papaya, banana or peeled pear; Eczema-Safe Fruit Salad, p. 246; or Healthy Skin Smoothie, p. 209 Filtered water and/or Healthy Skin Juice, p. 206	*Choose from:* papaya, banana or peeled pear; Eczema-Safe Fruit Salad, p. 246; or Healthy Skin Smoothie, p. 209 Filtered water and/or Healthy Skin Juice, p. 206	*Choose from:* papaya, banana or peeled pear; Eczema-Safe Fruit Salad, p. 246; or Healthy Skin Smoothie, p. 209 Filtered water and/or Healthy Skin Juice, p. 206	*Choose from:* Baked Banana Chips, p. 242; papaya, banana or peeled pear; Eczema-Safe Fruit Salad, p. 246; or Healthy Skin Smoothie, p. 209 Filtered water and/or Healthy Skin Juice, p. 206
Choose from: Design Your Own Sandwich, p. 223; Papaya Rice Paper Rolls, p. 222; Roasted Sweet Potato Salad, p. 219; or Roasted Potato Snack, p. 244 (all have GF options) Filtered water	*Choose from:* Design Your Own Sandwich, p. 223; Papaya Rice Paper Rolls, p. 222; Roasted Sweet Potato Salad, p. 219; or Roasted Potato Snack, p. 244 (all have GF options) Filtered water	*Choose from:* Design Your Own Sandwich, p. 223; Papaya Rice Paper Rolls, p. 222; Roasted Sweet Potato Salad, p. 219; or Roasted Potato Snack, p. 244 (all have GF options) Filtered water	*Choose from:* Spelt Lavash Bread, p. 243 with salad or Banana Carob Spread, p. 238; Design Your Own Sandwich, p. 223; Papaya Rice Paper Rolls, p. 222; or Roasted Potato Snack, p. 244 (all have GF options) Filtered water
Choose from: carrot and celery sticks with Sesame-Free Hummus, p. 239 and brown rice crackers; or Alkaline Bomb Salad, p. 218 Filtered water or Healthy Skin Juice, p. 206	*Choose from:* carrot and celery sticks with Sesame-Free Hummus, p. 239 and brown rice crackers; or Alkaline Bomb Salad, p. 218 Filtered water or Healthy Skin Juice, p. 206	*Choose from:* carrot and celery sticks with Sesame-Free Hummus, p. 239 and brown rice crackers; or Alkaline Bomb Salad, p. 218 Filtered water or Tarzan Juice, p. 207	*Choose from:* carrot and celery sticks with Sesame-Free Hummus, p. 239 and brown rice crackers; Alkaline Bomb Salad, p. 218; or Potato Wedges, p. 233 and Sesame-Free Hummus, p. 239 Filtered water or Healthy Skin Juice, p. 206
Choose from: Chicken Pasta with Green Beans, p. 230; or soup of choice, pp. 215–217	*Choose from:* My Favorite Lamb Chops, p. 231; or soup of choice, pp. 215–217 *Dessert:* papaya (rich in vitamin C to help iron absorption)	*Choose from:* Baked Fish with Mash, p. 225 (use eczema-safe white fish, p. 69); or soup of choice, pp. 215–217	*Choose from:* Easy Roast Chicken, p. 228; or soup of choice (V&Vn), pp. 215–217 *Optional Dessert:* Chocolate Milk, p. 210; Banana Icy Poles, p. 251; or Baked Banana Chips, p. 242
___/10	___/10	___/10	___/10

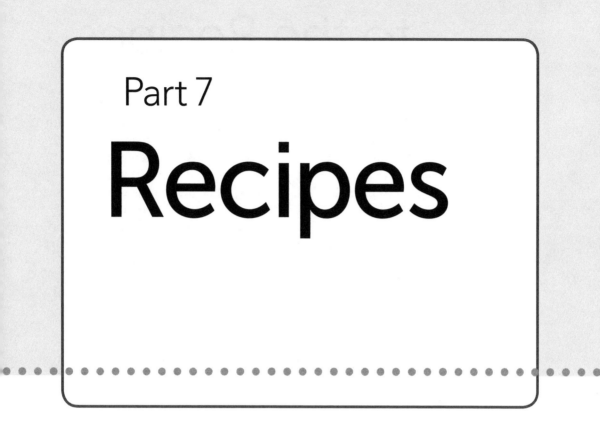

Part 7

Recipes

Introduction
to the Recipes

• •

In your kitchen, using specially selected ingredients, you can create delicious eczema-safe meals that can improve the health of your whole body. I encourage you to make these recipes your own and experiment with the eczema-safe ingredients.

Computer-assisted nutrient analysis of the recipes was prepared by Kimberly Zammit, HBSc (the project supervisor was Len Piché, PhD, RD, Division of Food & Nutritional Sciences, Brescia University College, London, ON), using Food Processor® SQL, version 10.9, ESHA Research Inc., Salem OR (this software contains over 35,000 food items based largely on the latest USDA data and the entire Canadian Nutrient File, 2007b). The database was supplemented when necessary with data from the Canadian Nutrient File (version 2010) and documented data from other reliable sources.

The analysis was based on:

- imperial weights and measures (except for foods typically packaged and used in metric quantities);
- the larger number of servings (i.e., the smaller portion) when there is a range;
- the smaller ingredient quantity when there was a range;
- the first ingredient listed when there was a choice of ingredients.

Calculations involving meat and poultry use lean portions without skin and with visible fat trimmed. A pinch of salt was calculated as $\frac{1}{8}$ tsp (0.5 mL). All recipes were analyzed prior to cooking. Optional ingredients and garnishes, and ingredients that are not quantified, were not included in the calculations.

All percent daily values (% DVs) and nutrition claims that appear in the recipes are based on U.S. standards.

Breakfast, Baby Food and Beverages

Omega Muesli

½ cup	rolled oats (see tip, at left)	125 mL
1 tsp	whole flax seeds	5 mL
	Filtered water	
	Sprinkle of ascorbic acid or citric acid (optional)	
	Soy milk or rice milk	
½	banana, sliced	½
1 tsp	soy lecithin granules (optional)	5 mL

Makes 1 serving

This tasty muesli is rich in omega-3s, vitamin C, potassium and fiber. Soaking the oats and flax seeds overnight with ascorbic acid (pure vitamin C) or citric acid reduces the phytic acid content and increases mineral availability.

1. Place oats and flax seeds in a bowl and add enough water to cover. If desired, add a sprinkle of ascorbic acid. Cover with plastic wrap and let stand overnight. (Do not refrigerate.)

2. The next morning, strain off the water and rinse the oats and seeds with plenty of filtered water. Transfer oats and seeds to a bowl, add soy milk and top with banana and lecithin granules (if using).

Tips

If making this for older children, reduce the oats to ⅓ cup (75 mL). For younger children, reduce the oats to ¼ cup (60 mL).

If you are allergic or sensitive to soy, omit the soy lecithin granules.

Variations

Use sliced pear or papaya instead of banana.

For Stage 2 only: Add a sprinkle of ground cinnamon before serving.

Health Tip

Although it is acceptable to use modern medicines to help you or your child gain temporary relief from eczema, a long-term solution involves dietary changes.

Nutrients per serving	
Calories	218

Total Fat
  Saturated Fat
  Omega-3
	5 g
	1 g
	0.6 g

Carbohydrate	42 g
Fiber	7 g (28% DV)
Protein	6 g
Biotin	3 mcg (1% DV)
Vitamin C	5 mg (8% DV)
Iron	2.1 mg (12% DV)
Magnesium	16 mg (4% DV)
Zinc	0 mg (0% DV)

Surprise Porridge

<table>
<tr><td></td></tr>
</table>

Makes 1 serving

For added omega-3 goodness, add whole or freshly ground flax seeds to this recipe before serving.

Tips

If making this for older children, reduce the oats to 1/3 cup (75 mL). For younger children, reduce the oats to 1/4 cup (60 mL).

If you are allergic or sensitive to soy, omit the soy lecithin granules.

Variation

For Stage 2 only: Add a sprinkle of ground cinnamon before serving.

1/2 cup	rolled oats (see tip, at left)	125 mL
	Filtered water	
	Sprinkle of ascorbic acid or citric acid (optional)	
	Fresh fruit (peeled pear, banana or papaya)	
	Soy milk or rice milk	
1 tsp	soy lecithin granules (optional)	5 mL

1. Place oats in a bowl and add enough water to cover. If desired, add a sprinkle of ascorbic acid. Cover with plastic wrap and let stand overnight. (Do not refrigerate.)

2. The next morning, strain off the water and rinse the oats with plenty of filtered water. Transfer oats to a saucepan with 1 1/2 cups (375 mL) filtered water (or 3 parts water to 1 part oats if using smaller amounts for children). Bring to a boil, then reduce heat and simmer, stirring occasionally, for 15 minutes.

3. Place fruit in a bowl (this is the surprise: the fruit is at the bottom). Pour in cooked oats and top with soy milk, soy lecithin (if using) and extra fruit, if desired.

Nutrients per serving	
Calories	255

Total Fat
    Saturated Fat
    Omega-3
	3 g
	1 g
	0.0 g

Carbohydrate	54 g
Fiber	7 g (28% DV)
Protein	6 g
Biotin	4 mcg (1% DV)
Vitamin C	10 mg (17% DV)
Iron	2.1 mg (12% DV)
Magnesium	32 mg (8% DV)
Zinc	0 mg (0% DV)

Quinoa Porridge

Quinoa is a nutritious, gluten-free grain for those who cannot eat oat porridge. Use red quinoa if available, as it is rich in skin-protective anthocyanins. It is optional to pre-soak the quinoa.

Tips

If making this for older children, reduce the quinoa to $1/3$ cup (75 mL). For younger children, reduce the quinoa to $1/4$ cup (60 mL).

To reduce the phytic acid content of flax seeds, soak them overnight.

To make this gluten-free, be sure to purchase malt-free soy milk or rice milk.

Variation

For Stage 2 only: Add a sprinkle of ground cinnamon before serving.

Nutrients per serving	
Calories	533

Total Fat
   Saturated Fat
   Omega-3
	9 g
	1 g
	1.0 g

Carbohydrate	101 g
Fiber	12 g (48% DV)
Protein	17 g
Biotin	7 mcg (2% DV)
Vitamin C	180 mg (300% DV)
Iron	5.6 mg (31% DV)
Magnesium	198 mg (50% DV)
Zinc	3 mg (20% DV)

$1/2$ cup	red or white quinoa, rinsed (do not use puffed quinoa)	125 mL
	Filtered water	
	Sprinkle of ascorbic acid or citric acid	
$1/2$ tsp	vanilla extract (optional)	2 mL
$1/2$ cup	soy milk or rice milk	125 mL
1 tsp	whole flax seeds (see tip, at left)	5 mL
1 tsp	rice malt syrup (optional)	5 mL
	Fresh fruit (papaya, banana or peeled pear)	

1. Place quinoa and 1 cup (250 mL) water in a bowl. Add a sprinkle of ascorbic or citric acid. Cover with plastic wrap and let stand overnight. (Do not refrigerate.)

2. The next morning, strain off the water and rinse the quinoa with plenty of filtered water. Transfer oats to a pot with $1\frac{1}{2}$ cups (375 mL) filtered water (or 3 parts water to 1 part oats if using smaller amounts for children). Bring to a boil, then reduce heat to low and cook until porridge is thick and grains are tender, about 20 minutes. Stir in vanilla and milk; cook for 5 minutes, stirring occasionally to prevent burning and adding more milk or water if necessary (you want lots of liquid to puff up the quinoa so it's very soft).

3. Serve with flax seeds, rice malt syrup (if using) and fruit.

Spelt Pancakes

<table>
<tr><td>Makes 6 to
8 pancakes</td></tr>
</table>

Spelt is easier to digest than wheat flour and provides a broader range of nutrients, including manganese, magnesium and copper, which are vital for healthy collagen production in the skin. Spelt pancakes taste very similar to wheat pancakes, and they are great for breakfast, dessert or a snack. The gluten-free version is Buckwheat Crêpes (page 202).

Tip

Turn the pancakes when the top starts to bubble.

Variations

For Stage 2 only: Add a sprinkle of ground cinnamon to the batter.

If you are allergic to soy, use rice milk in this recipe.

Nutrients per pancake	
Calories	97
Total Fat Saturated Fat Omega-3	2 g 0 g 0.0 g
Carbohydrate	17 g
Fiber	2 g (8% DV)
Protein	5 g
Biotin	7 mcg (2% DV)
Vitamin C	1 mg (2% DV)
Iron	0.9 mg (5% DV)
Magnesium	14 mg (4% DV)
Zinc	0 mg (0% DV)

1 cup	spelt flour, preferably whole-grain	250 mL
1/4 tsp	baking soda	1 mL
1 1/4 cups	soy milk	300 mL
1	egg, lightly beaten, or egg-free equivalent	1
	Rice bran oil	
	Rice malt syrup	
1 to 2	bananas, sliced (or 1/2 papaya, sliced)	1 to 2

1. In a bowl, combine spelt flour and baking soda (sift, if necessary). Gradually add milk, stirring until lump-free. Stir in egg.

2. In a small nonstick skillet, heat a little bit of oil over medium heat. Using a 1/3-cup (75 mL) measure, pour batter into the pan. Cook, turning once, until lightly browned on both sides. Transfer to a plate and keep warm. Repeat, adding more oil and adjusting heat as needed, until all the batter has been used.

3. Spread a thin layer of rice malt syrup on the pancakes and top with bananas.

Buckwheat Crêpes

| | Makes 8 to 10 crêpes | |

Buckwheat flour is an incredibly nutritious, grain-like flour with strong anti-inflammatory properties thanks to its rich content of antioxidants, including rutin, quercetin, zinc and selenium. It's also gluten-free and a good source of magnesium and manganese, which are vital for healthy collagen production in the skin. To make this meal gluten-free, use malt-free soy milk (rice milk can be used, but it does not work as well). Enjoy this meal for breakfast or as a healthy dessert.

Tip

Turn the crêpes when the top starts to bubble.

1 cup	buckwheat flour	250 mL
½ cup	brown rice flour	125 mL
½ tsp	baking soda	2 mL
2 cups	organic malt-free soy milk	500 mL
2	eggs, lightly beaten, or egg-free equivalent	2
½ tsp	vanilla extract (optional)	2 mL
	Rice bran oil	
	Rice malt syrup	
2	bananas, sliced	2

1. In a bowl, combine buckwheat flour, rice flour and baking soda (sift, if necessary). Gradually add milk, stirring until lump-free. Stir in eggs and vanilla.

2. In a small nonstick skillet, heat a little bit of oil over medium heat. Pour in a thin layer of batter and cook, turning once, until lightly browned on both sides. Transfer to a plate and keep warm. Repeat, adding more oil and adjusting heat as needed, until all the batter has been used.

3. Top each crêpe with rice malt syrup and sliced banana. Fold in half, if desired.

Health Tip

Although buckwheat flour is not as potent as quercetin, it supplies dietary fiber and is a nutritious way to add skin-repairing nutrients into your diet.

Nutrients per crêpe

Calories	104
Total Fat	2 g
Saturated Fat	0 g
Omega-3	0.0 g
Carbohydrate	18 g
Fiber	3 g (12% DV)
Protein	4 g
Biotin	5 mcg (2% DV)
Vitamin C	2 mg (3% DV)
Iron	0.8 mg (4% DV)
Magnesium	19 mg (5% DV)
Zinc	0 mg (0% DV)

Pear Muffins

Makes 12 muffins

Spelt flour makes muffins eczema-friendly and easier to digest than regular muffins, and they are ideal as a protein-rich snack, dessert or lunch box item. Spelt provides a broad range of nutrients, including manganese, magnesium and copper, which are vital for healthy collagen production.

Tips

If golden syrup is not available, use pure maple syrup or rice malt syrup (rice malt syrup is not as sweet).

Use real vanilla extract, not the imitation vanilla.

These muffins can be stored in an airtight container in the freezer for up to 3 months.

Nutrients per muffin	
Calories	186
Total Fat	7 g
Saturated Fat	1 g
Omega-3	0.1 g
Carbohydrate	29 g
Fiber	3 g (12% DV)
Protein	5 g
Biotin	1 mcg (2% DV)
Vitamin C	2 mg (3% DV)
Iron	1.1 mg (6% DV)
Magnesium	10 mg (3% DV)
Zinc	0 mg (0% DV)

- **Preheat oven to 350°F (180°C)**
- **Food processor**
- **Muffin pan, lined with paper liners or greased with rice bran oil**

1	egg or egg-free substitute	1
1/3 cup	golden syrup (see tip, at left)	75 mL
1 cup	soy milk or rice milk	250 mL
1/2 tsp	vanilla extract	2 mL
1/3 cup	rice bran oil	75 mL
2 cups	spelt flour, preferably whole-grain	500 mL
3 tsp	wheat-free baking powder	15 mL
1/2 tsp	baking soda	2 mL
2	large ripe pears, peeled and diced	2

1. In food processor, combine egg, golden syrup, milk and vanilla; process until smooth. With the motor running, slowly drizzle rice bran oil through the chute; process until smooth and creamy.

2. In a bowl, combine spelt flour, baking powder and baking soda (sift, if necessary). Add to the food processor and process briefly on low speed until combined. Using a spoon, gently stir in pear.

3. Spoon batter into prepared muffin cups, filling each three-quarters full.

4. Bake in preheated oven for 15 minutes or until light golden on top and a toothpick inserted in the center comes out clean. Let cool on a wire rack.

Variations

If you are gluten intolerant, try using an all-purpose gluten-free flour mix instead of the spelt flour; you may need a little less milk (use malt-free soy milk).

For Stage 2 only: Add a sprinkle of ground cinnamon to the batter and add a handful of blueberries when you stir in the pear.

Teething Rusks

<table>
<tr><td colspan="2">Makes about 20 rusks</td></tr>
</table>

Homemade teething rusks that are milk- and wheat-free are best for babies with eczema. You can experiment with this recipe and other ingredients to give your baby a variety of flavors and nutrients (see variation, below).

Tips

Make sure to cook the rusks until hard, so they don't break too easily when chewed.

When feeding your infant teething rusks, finger foods or any other food that could be a choking hazard, it's important to supervise your child and ensure that he or she is sitting upright.

Rusks can be stored in an airtight container at room temperature for up to 1 week.

Nutrients per rusk	
Calories	39
Total Fat	0 g
Saturated Fat	0 g
Omega-3	0.0 g
Carbohydrate	9 g
Fiber	1 g (4% DV)
Protein	1 g
Biotin	1 mcg (0% DV)
Vitamin C	1 mg (2% DV)
Iron	0.2 mg (1% DV)
Magnesium	12 mg (3% DV)
Zinc	0 mg (0% DV)

- **Preheat oven to 300°F (150°C)**
- **Food processor**
- **Baking sheets, lined with parchment paper**

1 cup	mashed banana	250 mL
1 cup	rice flour (brown, if available)	250 mL
	Filtered water	
	Rice flour for dusting	

1. In food processor, purée banana. Add rice flour and process on low speed until combined. Add water, if necessary, 1 tsp (5 mL) at a time, to make a stiff, dryish dough (do not make it wet).

2. On a floured surface, roll dough out into long, thin cylinders. Cut into 3-inch (7.5 cm) lengths. Place on prepared baking sheets.

3. Bake in preheated oven for 1 to 2 hours or until rusks are hard. Let cool completely on a wire rack.

Variation

Replace the banana with 1 cup (250 mL) mashed Stewed Pears (page 247) or any other eczema-safe fruit or vegetable, such as 1 cup (250 mL) cooked sweet potato, rutabaga or carrots.

Happy Face on Rice

Makes 2 servings for small children

You can adapt this basic, healthy children's lunch or dinner by adding cooked skinless chicken, lean lamb, fresh fish (see list, page 119), chickpeas or tofu for added protein. The red cabbage contains powerful anthocyanins that, if consumed frequently, can help protect your child's skin from UV sunlight.

Variation

For Stage 2 only: Add 1 tsp (5 mL) organic tomato ketchup — it is rich in skin-protective lycopene.

- **Steamer**

1 tbsp	Therapeutic Broth (page 212; optional)	15 mL
½ cup	warm cooked rice	125 mL
2	green beans (or 2 celery stalks, chopped)	2
2	slices red cabbage, cut into a smile shape	2
4	carrot slices	4
¼ cup	shredded cooked skinless chicken or other protein of choice	60 mL

1. If using Therapeutic Broth, mix it with the rice.

2. In a steamer, steam green beans, cabbage and carrots until soft.

3. Place rice in a bowl and arrange chicken and steamed vegetables to make a smiling face or a clock face.

Nutrients per serving	
Calories	98

Total Fat
  Saturated Fat
  Omega-3
	1 g
	0 g
	0.0 g

Carbohydrate	15 g
Fiber	2 g (8% DV)
Protein	7 g
Biotin	4 mcg (1% DV)
Vitamin C	15 mg (25% DV)
Iron	0.6 mg (3% DV)
Magnesium	36 mg (9% DV)
Zinc	1 mg (7% DV)

Healthy Skin Juice

Makes 2 servings

This highly alkalizing drink is designed to reduce inflammation, restore acid-alkaline balance in the body and aid liver detoxification of chemicals. It contains salicylates, so if you are highly sensitive, choose Tarzan Juice (page 207) instead. If available, use purple carrots, as they are rich in skin-protective anthocyanins.

- **Juicer**

3	stalks celery, scrubbed	3
1 to 2	carrots, scrubbed	1 to 2
½	medium beet, scrubbed	½
2	ripe pears, peeled	2
	Filtered water	

1. Using the juicer, juice celery, carrots, beet and pears. Add a splash of filtered water.

Variation

For Stage 2 only: Add a small knob of peeled gingerroot, as it has strong anti-inflammatory properties.

Health Tip

When introducing a new food, it is best to begin with small amounts only, because the overconsumption of one or two Stage 2 foods may cause flare-ups and dishearten you. If you are quite sensitive, you may like to begin by eating your favorite Stage 2 ingredients in small portions once a week and slowly build up to two or more times a week.

Nutrients per serving	
Calories	154
Total Fat	0 g
Saturated Fat	0 g
Omega-3	0.0 g
Carbohydrate	40 g
Fiber	9 g (36% DV)
Protein	2 g
Biotin	2 mcg (1% DV)
Vitamin C	13 mg (22% DV)
Iron	0.6 mg (3% DV)
Magnesium	26 mg (7% DV)
Zinc	0 mg (0% DV)

Tarzan Juice

This drink is designed to restore acid-alkaline balance in the body and aid liver detoxification of chemicals. Adjust the measurements to suit your tastes.

Tip

Sprouting mung beans is easy. See page 66 for instructions.

- **Juicer**

4	stalks celery, scrubbed	4
¼ to ½ cup	mung bean sprouts, washed	60 to 125 mL
2	large ripe pears, peeled	2
	Filtered water	

1. Using the juicer, juice celery, sprouts and pears. Add a splash of filtered water.

Variation

Add a handful of fresh parsley with the pears.

Nutrients per serving	
Calories	149
Total Fat	0 g
Saturated Fat	0 g
Omega-3	0.0 g
Carbohydrate	39 g
Fiber	9 g (36% DV)
Protein	2 g
Biotin	1 mcg (0% DV)
Vitamin C	14 mg (23% DV)
Iron	0.7 mg (6% DV)
Magnesium	28 mg (7% DV)
Zinc	0 mg (0% DV)

Flaxseed Lemon Drink

<table>
<tr><td>

Makes 2 servings

</td></tr>
</table>

This is a Stage 2 recipe. Over the years, I've had such great feedback about this alkalizing drink. The oils from the lemon zest provide antioxidants, chelate toxins from the bowel and stimulate liver detoxification enzymes. The lecithin aids fat digestion and helps the body use the anti-inflammatory omega-3 oil. A word of caution: this drink is only suitable for those who are not sensitive to salicylates or amines, as lemon is rich in both.

Tip

Enjoy this drink throughout the day or before each main meal.

* **Blender**

	Finely grated zest and juice of ½ lemon	
2 cups	chilled filtered water	500 mL
1 tbsp	soy lecithin granules	15 mL
2 tsp	organic flaxseed oil	10 mL

1. In blender, combine lemon zest, lemon juice, water, soy lecithin and flaxseed oil. Blend on high for 30 seconds or until frothy. Strain, if desired.

Nutrients per serving	
Calories	73

Total Fat
  Saturated Fat
  Omega-3
	7 g
	1 g
	2.4 g

Carbohydrate	1 g
Fiber	0 g (0% DV)
Protein	0 g
Biotin	0 mcg (0% DV)
Vitamin C	5 mg (8% DV)
Iron	0.2 mg (1% DV)
Magnesium	3 mg (1% DV)
Zinc	0 mg (0% DV)

Healthy Skin Smoothie

Makes 2 servings

This drink is designed to calm the itch of eczema and hydrate the skin. Pre-freeze a peeled banana to make this smoothie cold.

Variations

You can add 1 sprig of fresh parsley for alkalizing.

For Stage 2 only: Add a sprinkle of ground cinnamon.

- **Blender**

1	frozen ripe banana, chopped	1
1	slice papaya, chopped	1
1½ cups	chilled soy milk or rice milk	375 mL
1 tbsp	soy lecithin granules	15 mL
1 tsp	flaxseed oil or ground flax seeds	5 mL
Dash	vanilla extract (optional)	Dash

1. In blender, combine banana, papaya, soy milk, soy lecithin, flaxseed oil and vanilla (if using). Blend on high speed until smooth.

Health Tip

If you are allergic to cinnamon, avoid it and test nutmeg instead (nutmeg also helps with blood sugar control). Buy whole nutmeg and finely grate it onto your breakfast cereals or use it whenever you use rice milk.

Nutrients per serving	
Calories	271

Total Fat
  Saturated Fat
  Omega-3
	8 g
	1 g
	1.4 g

Carbohydrate	44 g
Fiber	5 g (20% DV)
Protein	7 g
Biotin	12 mcg (4% DV)
Vitamin C	95 mg (158% DV)
Iron	1.9 mg (11% DV)
Magnesium	62 mg (16% DV)
Zinc	0 mg (0% DV)

Chocolate Milk (Hot or Cold)

<table>
<tr><td>Makes 1 to
2 servings</td></tr>
</table>

**Makes 1 to
2 servings**

This tasty carob drink is caffeine-free and is suitable as an occasional treat.

1 tsp	carob powder	5 mL
1½ cups	soy milk or rice milk	375 mL
1 tsp	rice malt syrup (optional)	5 mL

Cold Chocolate Milk

1. The secret to a lump-free drink is to mix the carob powder in 2 tsp (10 mL) boiling hot water before adding it to the soy milk. Taste and sweeten with rice malt syrup if desired. (Alternatively, combine all ingredients in a blender and blend on high speed until smooth.)

Hot Chocolate

1. In a small saucepan, heat soy milk over medium heat until warm (or hot, if desired). Stir in carob powder and rice malt syrup (if using).

Nutrients per 1 of 2 servings	
Calories	102

Total Fat
  Saturated Fat
  Omega-3
	3 g
	0 g
	0.1 g

Carbohydrate	12 g
Fiber	1 g (4% DV)
Protein	6 g
Biotin	10 mcg (3% DV)
Vitamin C	0 mg (0% DV)
Iron	1.2 mg (7% DV)
Magnesium	46 mg (12% DV)
Zinc	0 mg (0% DV)

Soups
and Salads

Therapeutic Broth

Makes 6 to 8 cups (1.5 to 2 L)

This alkaline broth is rich in glycine, collagen, calcium and magnesium. It boosts liver detoxification, heals the digestive tract and can reduce inflammation and strengthen the immune system. The secret to a therapeutic broth is the addition of a weak acid, such as citric acid or ascorbic acid (pure vitamin C), to draw out the minerals from the bones. Drink this broth daily: 1/2 cup (125 mL) for adults, 1/4 cup (60 mL) for children and 1 to 2 tsp (5 to 10 mL) for infants over 4 months. Omit the salt for infants or people with high blood pressure. It also makes a tasty stock for casseroles and soups.

Nutrients per 1 cup (250 mL)	
Calories	60

Total Fat
  Saturated Fat
  Omega-3
	1 g
	0.5 g
	0.0 g

Carbohydrate	10 g
Fiber	2 g (8% DV)
Protein	4 g
Biotin	2 mcg (1% DV)
Vitamin C	14 mg (23% DV)
Iron	1 mg (6% DV)
Magnesium	20 mg (5% DV)
Zinc	0 mg (0% DV)

- **Preheat oven to 400°F (200°C)**
- **Roasting pan**

2	large beef bones, with a little meat on them (including necks, joints, marrow, lamb bones)	2
14 cups	filtered water, at room temperature	3.5 L
1	large free-range organic chicken carcass (or 2 small)	1
1/4 tsp	ascorbic acid or citric acid	1 mL
1	large leek (white part only)	1
2	green onions, trimmed	2
2	Brussels sprouts	2
2	stalks celery	2
1	potato (with skin)	1
2	cloves garlic, minced	2
1 tsp	sea salt, preferably Celtic (optional)	5 mL

1. In roasting pan, roast beef bones in preheated oven for 30 minutes or until fragrant and browned. Transfer to a stockpot or very large saucepan and add water, chicken carcass and ascorbic acid. Cover and bring to a boil. Reduce heat to low and simmer for 1 to 2 hours.

2. Meanwhile, scrub and chop the leek, green onions, Brussels sprouts, celery and potato into small pieces.

3. Using tongs, break apart the carcasses to allow more minerals to be extracted from the bones. Add chopped vegetables, garlic and salt (if using). Cook for 4 to 5 hours or until broth is reduced by almost half.

Tips

Step 5 is very important, so don't be tempted to skip it.

If your broth is thick and jelly-like, it means it's rich in collagen (gelatin).

Broth will last for 1 week in the refrigerator. Store broth in clean glass jars or airtight containers, and freeze the leftovers. Most soup or casserole recipes use 3 cups (750 mL) of broth, so measure portions of 3 cups (750 mL) each and write the volume on the container before freezing. Freeze 1-tbsp (15 mL) portions in ice cube trays for use in pasta dishes or children's meals.

4. Remove bones (chicken bones should be soft and should crumble when squeezed). Place a strainer over a large bowl, then pour broth through the strainer, discarding the bones and vegetables. Squeeze out as much liquid as possible as you strain the broth (use a measuring cup and press on the cooked meat and vegetables to squeeze out the liquid).

5. Store the broth in an airtight container in the refrigerator overnight so the fat has time to solidify. The next day, carefully lift or skim off the layer of fat (this saturated fat is no good for your eczema).

Health Tip

A well-made broth soothes the gastrointestinal tract and provides the skin-repairing amino acid glycine. Glycine is needed to produce connective tissue and enhances detoxification of chemicals. Broth contains collagen, calcium, and magnesium, and for those in poor health or suffering from a cold or flu, sipping cysteine-rich broth throughout the day can reduce mucus and offer relief.

Alkaline Veggie Broth

This nutritious alkaline vegan broth is rich in flavonoids and anti-oxidants. Use it to flavor soups and casseroles.

Tip

Broth will last for 1 week in the refrigerator. Store broth in clean glass jars or airtight containers, and freeze the leftovers. Most soup or casserole recipes use 3 cups (750 m) of broth, so measure portions of 3 cups (750 mL) each and write the volume on the container before freezing. Freeze 1-tbsp (15 mL) portions in ice cube trays for use in pasta dishes or children's meals.

Variation

For Stage 2 only: Add 1/2 tsp (2 mL) grated gingerroot and 1 bay leaf.

Nutrients per 1 cup (250 mL)	
Calories	72
Total Fat	0 g
Saturated Fat	0 g
Omega-3	0.2 g
Carbohydrate	16 g
Fiber	3 g (12% DV)
Protein	2 g
Biotin	2 mcg (1% DV)
Vitamin C	29 mg (48% DV)
Iron	1.1 mg (6% DV)
Magnesium	25 mg (6% DV)
Zinc	0 mg (0% DV)

1	leek (white part only), finely sliced	1
2	cloves garlic, minced	2
10 cups	filtered water	2.5 L
3	stalks celery, chopped	3
3	Brussels sprouts, chopped	3
3	potatoes (with skin), scrubbed and diced	3
1	handful fresh parsley	1
1 tsp	sea salt, preferably Celtic	5 mL
Pinch	ascorbic acid (optional)	Pinch

1. In a stockpot or very large saucepan, heat a splash of filtered water over medium heat. Sauté leek and garlic for 5 minutes. Add water, celery, Brussels sprouts, potatoes, parsley, salt and ascorbic acid (if using); cover and bring to a boil.

2. Reduce heat to low and simmer, stirring occasionally, for 1 to 2 hours. Remove from heat and let cool for a few minutes. Strain the broth, using a spatula or measuring cup to press the liquid from the vegetables. Discard the strained vegetables.

New Potato and Leek Soup

<table>
<tr><td>

Makes 6 to 8 servings

</td></tr>
</table>

This smooth, alkalizing soup is rich in skin-protective antioxidants. Leeks supply vitamin K and anti-inflammatory quercetin, and potatoes are a good source of dietary fiber, vitamin C, choline, iron, potassium, manganese and vitamin B6, which are essential for healthy skin. It's best to use new potatoes, as they have a lower GI rating, but if they are unavailable in your area, any variety of white potato is fine.

Tip

Add more water to leftover soup the next day if it thickens overnight.

* **Blender or food processor**

2	large leeks (white parts only), finely sliced	2
2	cloves garlic, minced	2
3 cups	Therapeutic Broth (page 212) or Alkaline Veggie Broth (page 214)	750 mL
6 cups	filtered water	1.5 L
2½ lbs	new potatoes, peeled and chopped	1.25 kg
4	Brussels sprouts, diced	4
¼ cup	fresh parsley leaves, chopped	60 mL
½ tsp	sea salt, preferably Celtic (optional)	2 mL

1. In a stockpot or very large saucepan, heat a splash of filtered water over medium heat. Lightly sauté leeks and garlic. Add broth and water; cover and bring to a boil.

2. Add potatoes and Brussels sprouts; cover and bring to a boil. Reduce heat to low and simmer, stirring occasionally, for 20 to 30 minutes or until potatoes are tender. Remove from heat, uncover and let cool for 5 minutes. Stir in parsley and salt.

3. One batch at a time, process soup in blender until smooth. The soup should have a thick consistency. If it's too thick, add more water.

Nutrients per 1 of 8 servings	
Calories	155

Total Fat
  Saturated Fat
  Omega-3
	0 g
	0 g
	0.1 g

Carbohydrate	35 g
Fiber	5 g (20% DV)
Protein	5 g
Biotin	4 mcg (1% DV)
Vitamin C	53 mg (88% DV)
Iron	2.3 mg (13% DV)
Magnesium	53 mg (13% DV)
Zinc	1 mg (7% DV)

Sunshine Soup

This smooth, alkalizing soup is designed to boost the immune system and soothe the digestive tract. Sweet potato is an excellent source of dietary fiber, carotenes (vitamin A), vitamin C, vitamin B6, magnesium and manganese, which are essential for healthy skin.

Tip

Sweet potato contains moderate salicylates. For fewer salicylates, use 2 sweet potatoes and 5 medium potatoes (peeled).

- **Blender or food processor**

3 cups	Therapeutic Broth (page 212) or Alkaline Veggie Broth (page 214)	750 mL
4 cups	filtered water (approx.)	1 L
2½ lbs	sweet potatoes (about 4 large), peeled and chopped	1.25 kg
2	cloves garlic, minced	2
1	leek (white part only), finely chopped	1
	Sea salt, preferably Celtic (optional)	
1	handful chopped fresh parsley (optional)	1

1. In a stockpot or large saucepan, combine broth and water; cover and bring to a boil. Add sweet potatoes, garlic and leek; reduce heat to low, cover and simmer for 25 minutes. Season to taste with salt, if desired. Remove from heat and let cool for 5 minutes.

2. One batch at a time, process soup in blender until smooth, adding another ½ cup (125 mL) or more water if necessary. Serve garnished with parsley, if desired.

Nutrients per serving	
Calories	190

Total Fat
  Saturated Fat
  Omega-3
	1 g
	0 g
	0.0 g

Carbohydrate	44 g
Fiber	6 g (24% DV)
Protein	4 g
Biotin	10 mcg (3% DV)
Vitamin C	41 mg (68% DV)
Iron	2.2 mg (12% DV)
Magnesium	53 mg (13% DV)
Zinc	1 mg (7% DV)

Country Chicken Soup

This classic chicken soup is rich in inflammation-lowering antioxidants and contains Therapeutic Broth, which boosts the immune system. Barley is a low-GI carbohydrate that supplies dietary fiber and promotes a healthy digestive tract. If you cannot eat gluten, replace the barley with ¼ cup (60 mL) red quinoa or rice. You can also adapt this recipe by using eczema-safe fish or cooked beans instead of chicken.

3 cups	Therapeutic Broth (page 212) or Alkaline Veggie Broth (page 214)	750 mL
6 cups	filtered water	1.5 L
2	cloves garlic, minced	2
1	large carrot, finely diced	1
2	stalks celery, cut lengthwise and finely diced	2
1	small leek (white part only), finely chopped	2
2	Brussels sprouts, finely diced	2
½ cup	barley, rinsed, preferably soaked overnight (see page 76)	125 mL
¼ to ½ tsp	sea salt, preferably Celtic (optional)	1 to 2 mL
14 oz	boneless skinless chicken breasts or thighs, finely diced	400 g

1. In a stockpot or large saucepan, combine broth and water; cover and bring to a boil. Add garlic, carrot, celery, leek, Brussels sprouts, barley and salt to taste (if using); reduce heat to low, cover and simmer for 25 minutes (45 minutes if barley has not been soaked). Add chicken and cook for 5 minutes or until no longer pink inside.

Variations

Garnish soup with chopped parsley.

Add extra vegetables if a heartier soup is desired.

For Stage 2 only: Add a sprinkle of grated gingerroot and a heaping teaspoon (5 mL) organic vegetable stock powder, if desired.

Nutrients per serving	
Calories	192
Total Fat Saturated Fat Omega-3	2 g 0.5 g 0.1 g
Carbohydrate	26 g
Fiber	5 g (20% DV)
Protein	18 g
Biotin	4 mcg (1% DV)
Vitamin C	25 mg (42% DV)
Iron	1.7 mg (9% DV)
Magnesium	53 mg (13% DV)
Zinc	1 mg (7% DV)

Alkaline Bomb Salad

Makes 2 servings

This salad contains highly alkalizing sprouts and vegetables to help restore acid-alkaline balance to the body, and it's topped with a tasty protein-rich dip. If serving to children, omit the green onions and serve each salad in an iceberg lettuce leaf "cup."

4	handfuls iceberg or romaine lettuce, torn	4
1	small stalk celery, chopped	1
1 to 2	green onions, thinly sliced on the diagonal	1 to 2
¼ to ½ cup	mung bean sprouts, washed	60 to 125 mL
3 tbsp	Sesame-Free Hummus (page 239) or Bean Dip (page 240)	45 mL

1. Divide lettuce between two shallow serving bowls. Top with celery, green onions and bean sprouts. Top each with a large dollop of hummus.

Health Tip

Mung bean sprouts are one of the few strongly alkalizing foods available. They contain magnesium, vitamin K, folate, potassium, and vitamin C, and they are salicylate-free.

Nutrients per serving	
Calories	45

Total Fat
  Saturated Fat
  Omega-3
	1 g
	0 g
	0.1 g

Carbohydrate	8 g
Fiber	3 g (12% DV)
Protein	3 g
Biotin	10 mcg (3% DV)
Vitamin C	10 mg (17% DV)
Iron	1.9 mg (11% DV)
Magnesium	19 mg (5% DV)
Zinc	0 mg (0% DV)

Roasted Sweet Potato Salad

Makes 2 servings

Salads help restore the body's acid-alkaline balance, and mung bean sprouts are highly alkalizing. Sweet potato is an excellent source of dietary fiber, carotenes (vitamin A), vitamin C, vitamin B6, magnesium and manganese. Hummus and cashews supply protein for a complete healthy skin meal.

Variation

For Stage 2 only: Add a teaspoon (5 mL) of Omega Salad Dressing (page 220) if you are not sensitive to sulfites (see apple cider vinegar information, page 172).

- **Preheat oven to 400°F (200°C)**
- **Rimmed baking sheet**

1	medium sweet potato, peeled and diced	1
½ tsp	rice bran oil	2 mL
	Sea salt, preferably Celtic	
3 cups	romaine or iceberg lettuce, torn	750 mL
3 tbsp	Sesame-Free Hummus (page 239)	45 mL
¼ cup	mung bean sprouts, washed	60 mL
	Unsalted raw cashews (optional)	

1. Lightly drizzle the sweet potato with rice bran oil (do not let the potato sit in oil) and sprinkle with salt. Spread out in a single layer on baking sheet. Roast in preheated oven for 30 minutes or until very tender.

2. Divide lettuce between two plates. Top with sweet potato and a large dollop of hummus. Sprinkle with sprouts and cashews (if using).

Nutrients per serving	
Calories	94

Total Fat
  Saturated Fat
  Omega-3
	2 g
	0 g
	0.1 g

Carbohydrate	17 g
Fiber	4 g (16% DV)
Protein	3 g
Biotin	12 mcg (4% DV)
Vitamin C	14 mg (23% DV)
Iron	1.7 mg (9% DV)
Magnesium	14 mg (4% DV)
Zinc	0 mg (0% DV)

Omega Salad Dressing

1 tbsp	rice bran oil	15 mL
2 tsp	flaxseed oil (see tip, at left)	10 mL
4 tsp	apple cider vinegar	20 mL
2 tbsp	rice malt syrup	30 mL

Makes about ⅓ cup (75 mL)

This dressing is highly alkalizing and makes a delicious addition to salads, but it's only recommended for Stage 2, as the apple cider vinegar may cause an adverse reaction in sensitive individuals. See "Other Stage 2 Additions" (page 171) for more information on apple cider vinegar.

Tips

Flaxseed oil changes the taste of the dressing, so adjust the amount to suit your palate.

Do not use flaxseed oil on hot foods, as heat damages the oil.

Variation

Add freshly minced garlic.

1. Place rice bran oil, flaxseed oil, vinegar and rice malt syrup into a jar and shake well.

2. Store in an airtight container in the refrigerator. Apple cider vinegar is a natural preservative, and the dressing will stay fresh for a few weeks if refrigerated. Use 1 tsp (5 mL) per person on salads or baked sweet potato recipes.

Health Tip

Although most vinegars are strongly acid-forming and unsuitable for eczema sufferers, apple cider vinegar is highly alkalizing and it can be beneficial for eczema. There is a catch, however. Apple cider vinegar is rich in natural chemicals, including sulfites, salicylates, and moderate amines, so it may cause your eczema to return, especially if you are sensitive to sulfites (if you have sulfite allergy, do not test apple cider vinegar).

Nutrients per 1 tsp (5 mL)	
Calories	24
Total Fat	2 g
Saturated Fat	0 g
Omega-3	0.3 g
Carbohydrate	3 g
Fiber	0 g (0% DV)
Protein	0 g
Biotin	0 mcg (0% DV)
Vitamin C	0 mg (0% DV)
Iron	0.0 mg (0% DV)
Magnesium	0 mg (0% DV)
Zinc	0 mg (0% DV)

Lunch and Dinner

Papaya Rice Paper Rolls

Makes 4 servings

Rice paper rolls make a healthy snack or a light meal. Use chicken, lean lamb or canned tuna (in water). There is no need to add sauce, as the papaya gives them a juicy burst of sweetness when you bite into them.

Variation

For Stage 2 only: Add chopped fresh mint.

- **Steamer**

1 lb	boneless skinless chicken, thinly sliced	500 g
	Minced garlic or garlic powder	
	Sea salt, preferably Celtic (optional)	
20	round rice papers	20
½	ripe papaya, thinly sliced	½
3	handfuls romaine or iceberg lettuce, finely shredded	3
2	medium carrots, grated	2
¾ cup	mung bean sprouts, washed	175 mL

1. Sprinkle chicken with garlic and salt. In a steamer, steam chicken for 5 minutes or until no longer pink inside. Remove from heat and let cool slightly.

2. Wet a clean tea towel, wring out excess water and place flat on the counter. Soften rice paper, one sheet at a time, in a large bowl of very warm water, soaking each one for 10 to 20 seconds or according to the package instructions. Remove rice paper before it gets too soft and place flat on the damp tea towel.

3. Working with one piece of rice paper, arrange chicken, papaya, lettuce, carrots and bean sprouts in a row near the end closest to you. Roll rice paper up, tucking the ends in about halfway through, to form a cylinder.

Nutrients per serving	
Calories	351

Total Fat
   Saturated Fat
   Omega-3
	4 g
	 1 g
	 0.0 g

Carbohydrate	44 g
Fiber	2 g (8% DV)
Protein	34 g
Biotin	7 mcg (2% DV)
Vitamin C	35 mg (58% DV)
Iron	1.4 mg (8% DV)
Magnesium	40 mg (10% DV)
Zinc	1 mg (7% DV)

Design Your Own Sandwich

Eczema-safe sandwiches and wraps are great for lunches and snacks. Here are your options.

Bread Choices
- Spelt sourdough (available from some health food shops)
- Spelt tortillas (make sure they are free of artificial additives)
- Spelt Lavash Bread (page 243)
- Gluten-free bread (make sure the ingredients are all or mostly eczema-safe)
- Multigrain or whole-grain rye crispbread (make sure there are no trans fats)

Spread Choices
- Banana Carob Spread (page 238)
- Sesame-Free Hummus (page 239)
- Bean Dip (page 240)
- Parsley Pesto (page 241; in moderation, not daily)
- Pure organic butter (for Stage 2 only and allergy permitting)

Filling Choices
- Cooked skinless chicken with mung bean sprouts
- Cooked skinless chicken with roasted potatoes
- Trout, salmon or tuna with grated carrot and iceberg lettuce
- Canned tuna with roasted sweet potato and romaine lettuce
- Home-cooked or organic turkey breast with romaine lettuce
- Sliced lean roast lamb with leftover roast vegetables
- Iceberg lettuce, mung bean sprouts, grated carrot and grated beets
- Banana and rice malt syrup (occasionally)
- Mashed boiled egg and iceberg lettuce (allergy permitting and preferably in Stage 2)

Tip
Use only organic or home-cooked meats. Pre-sliced meats and deli meats contain flavor enhancers and may contain irritating preservatives, such as nitrates.

Chickpea Casserole

Makes 6 servings

This dish is highly alkalizing and is designed to promote detoxification and reduce acid in the body. Chickpeas are a good source of protein, iron and manganese, which are essential for collagen production in the skin. Omit the flour if making this recipe for the 3-Day Alkalizing Cleanse.

- **Preheat oven to 350°F (180°C)**
- **Large casserole dish**

3 cups	Therapeutic Broth (page 212) or Alkaline Veggie Broth (page 214)	750 mL
1 cup	filtered water (or additional broth)	250 mL
1 to 2 tsp	brown rice flour or spelt flour	5 to 10 mL
2 cups	cooked chickpeas (or one 14-oz/398 mL cans chickpeas, drained and rinsed)	500 mL
4	potatoes, scrubbed and diced	4
1	medium sweet potato, peeled and diced	1
1	leek, finely chopped	1
3	Brussels sprouts, finely sliced	3
4	stalks celery, halved lengthwise and finely chopped	4
2	cloves garlic, minced	2
	Chopped parsley (optional)	
	Green onions (optional)	

1. Pour broth and water into casserole dish. In a cup, mix flour with a little water until there are no lumps, then stir into the broth. Add chickpeas, potatoes, sweet potato, leek, Brussels sprouts, celery and garlic.

2. Bake in preheated oven, stirring occasionally, for 1 hour. The casserole should be slightly soupy, so add more water if necessary. If desired, garnish with parsley or green onions.

Variations

Use skinless chicken instead of chickpeas, and add chopped green onions and rutabaga to the casserole. (During the 3-Day Alkalizing Cleanse, don't use chicken.)

For Stage 2 only: Add a little organic stock powder to see if you can tolerate it (it may contain salicylates and natural MSG). If you tolerate it well and don't have eczema, you can use a quality, all-natural stock powder and water instead of the broth when you are short on time.

For Stage 2 only: Add a sprinkle of ground cinnamon and/or cumin if you have tested them and tolerate them well.

Nutrients per serving	
Calories	159
Total Fat 　Saturated Fat 　Omega-3	1 g 0 g 0.0 g
Carbohydrate	33 g
Fiber	6 g (24% DV)
Protein	6 g
Biotin	14 mcg (5% DV)
Vitamin C	38 mg (63% DV)
Iron	2.2 mg (12% DV)
Magnesium	28 mg (7% DV)
Zinc	0 mg (0% DV)

Baked Fish with Mash

> **Makes 2 adult and 2 child-size servings**

Trout is rich in omega-3s, vitamin B_{12}, manganese, selenium and vitamin B_3. Here, it's teamed with alkalizing vegetables for an acid-alkaline-balanced meal.

Tips

Each serving of fish should be around the size of the palm of your hand. Fish is usually sold in large pieces, so you will probably only need half of one fillet per adult.

If the fish develops white clumps on the sides during cooking, it is overcooking. Remove it immediately from the oven.

Nutrients per adult serving

Calories	378
Total Fat	8 g
Saturated Fat	2 g
Omega-3	0.5 g
Carbohydrate	60 g
Fiber	12 g (48% DV)
Protein	18 g
Biotin	16 mcg (6% DV)
Vitamin C	94 mg (156% DV)
Iron	4.6 mg (26% DV)
Magnesium	76 mg (20% DV)
Zinc	1 mg (7% DV)

- **Preheat oven to 350°F (180°C)**
- **Steamer**
- **Baking dish, lined with parchment paper**

1	medium sweet potato, peeled and diced	1
3	potatoes, peeled and diced	3
	Splash of soy milk	
	Sea salt, preferably Celtic (optional)	
2	boneless trout fillets (see tip, at left), halved lengthwise	2
	Rice bran oil	
1	small handful flat-leaf (Italian) parsley, washed and chopped, stems removed	1
	Garlic powder	
3	handfuls green beans, ends trimmed	3
1½ cups	chopped red cabbage	375 mL

1. In a steamer, over a little water, steam sweet potato and potato for 15 minutes or until very soft (reserve the water for steaming the greens). Mash the potatoes, adding soy milk as needed (you may need up to $1/4$ cup/60 mL). Sprinkle with salt, if desired. Set aside.

2. Place fish in prepared baking dish. Lightly coat fish with rice bran oil and top with parsley and garlic powder.

3. Bake in preheated oven for 8 to 10 minutes or until fish is opaque and flakes easily when tested with a fork.

4. Meanwhile, steam the green beans and red cabbage until tender.

5. Reheat the mash before serving alongside trout and steamed vegetables.

Variations

If you are vegetarian or vegan, use tofu or cooked lentils, chickpeas or beans instead of fish. Steam the tofu along with the beans and cabbage. To cook legumes, see page 82.

For a gluten-free meal, use malt-free soy milk, rice milk or Therapeutic Broth (page 212) in the mash.

Sticks and Stones
(Fish or Chicken on Skewers)

<table>
<tr><td>

**Makes 2 adult
and 2 child-size
servings**

</td></tr>
</table>

Bamboo skewers are a creative way to present fish or chicken (or tofu if you are vegetarian or vegan). The bamboo skewers need to be soaked for at least 15 minutes to prevent them from burning during cooking.

Tip

For a heartier meal, serve with cooked basmati rice or brown rice. Do not use instant rice. Brown rice usually has a high glycemic index, so choose a low-GI variety if available or use basmati rice if you have blood sugar issues, such as diabetes.

Nutrients per adult serving	
Calories	304

Total Fat
   Saturated Fat
   Omega-3
	12 g
	2 g
	1.8 g

Carbohydrate	8 g
Fiber	2 g (8% DV)
Protein	40 g
Biotin	12 mcg (4% DV)
Vitamin C	16 mg (26% DV)
Iron	2.2 mg (12% DV)
Magnesium	64 mg (16% DV)
Zinc	1 mg (7% DV)

- **Preheat broiler**
- **12 to 14 bamboo skewers, soaked**

1¼ lbs	boneless trout fillets or boneless skinless chicken thighs	625 g
3	large green onions, cut into ¾-inch (2 cm) pieces	3
	Garlic powder	
	Fine sea salt, preferably Celtic (optional)	
	Alkaline Bomb Salad (page 218)	

1. Cut trout into ¾-inch (2 cm) cubes. Thread trout (or chicken) and green onions alternately onto skewers, leaving a 2-inch (5 cm) space at the blunt end of each skewer. Season with garlic powder and salt.

2. Broil for 5 minutes, turning once, until fish is opaque and flakes easily when tested with a fork (if using chicken, broil for at least 10 minutes or until juices run clear when chicken is pierced).

3. Serve skewers alongside Alkaline Bomb Salad.

Variation

If you are vegetarian or vegan, use firm tofu in place of the fish.

Cinnamon Chicken

Makes 2 adult and 2 child-size servings

Cinnamon is a delicious spice with strong antibacterial properties, and I recommend that you add this important ingredient to your diet during Stage 2. Cinnamon contains protective phytochemicals such as cinnamaldehyde, which reduces blood sugar levels, promotes satiety (so you're less likely to overeat) and lowers LDL cholesterol. If using this recipe during Stage 1, omit the cinnamon and use Celtic sea salt and dried parsley instead.

- **Steamer**

1 lb	boneless skinless chicken thighs, halved and fat removed	500 g
1 tsp	rice bran oil	5 mL
2	cloves garlic, minced	2
½ tsp	ground cinnamon	2 mL
5	green onions, chopped	5
4	large potatoes, scrubbed and chopped	4
1	small-medium sweet potato, peeled and chopped	1
1 cup	chopped red cabbage	250 mL
6	Brussels sprouts, finely sliced (or use green beans)	6
	Sea salt, preferably Celtic (optional)	

1. To promote even cooking, pound the chicken flat (do this in a plastic bag to prevent splattering). In a bowl, combine rice bran oil, garlic and cinnamon. Stir in chicken.

2. In a wok or large nonstick skillet, over medium-high heat, stir-fry chicken until no longer pink inside, adding green onions for the last 1 to 2 minutes of cooking.

3. Meanwhile, steam potatoes, sweet potato, cabbage and Brussels sprouts until soft. Sprinkle with sea salt if desired.

Nutrients per adult serving	
Calories	482
Total Fat Saturated Fat Omega-3	8 g 2 g 0.2 g
Carbohydrate	66 g
Fiber	10 g (40% DV)
Protein	38 g
Biotin	10 mcg (3% DV)
Vitamin C	116 mg (194% DV)
Iron	5.4 mg (30% DV)
Magnesium	120 mg (30% DV)
Zinc	4 mg (26% DV)

Easy Roast Chicken

Makes 6 servings

Serve this meal with Eczema-Safe Gravy (opposite). If available, use purple carrots, as they are rich in skin-protective anthocyanins.

Tips

You can steam the root veggies instead of roasting them, if you prefer.

Use leftover chicken meat to make Country Chicken Soup (page 217).

- **Preheat oven to 350°F (180°C)**
- **Large, deep baking pan with a wire rack**
- **Rimmed baking sheet, lined with parchment paper**
- **Steamer**

4 lb	whole chicken	2 kg
	Rice bran oil	
	Sea salt, preferably Celtic	
	Garlic powder	
8	potatoes (with skin), cut into chunks	8
4	carrots, sliced on the diagonal	4
½	sweet potato, peeled and sliced	½
4	Brussels sprouts	4
2	handfuls green beans, ends trimmed	2
1 cup	chopped red cabbage	250 mL

1. Rinse chicken inside and out. Pat the outside dry with a paper towel. Rub rice bran oil over the chicken, then sprinkle with salt and garlic powder. Place chicken upside down on rack in baking pan. (For an extra-tender roast, pour 1 cup/250 mL water into the bottom of the pan, ensuring the water does not touch the chicken.) Roast in preheated oven for 30 minutes.

2. Meanwhile, place potatoes, carrots and sweet potato in a large bowl. Drizzle with a little oil. Using a slotted spoon, transfer veggies to prepared baking sheet and sprinkle with salt (if more space is needed, some of the veggies can cook beside the chicken on the wire rack).

3. Turn chicken right side up and add the tray of veggies to the oven. Roast for 1 hour, turning veggies regularly, until chicken is no longer pink inside (check around the drumsticks by gently pulling the flesh away from the bone).

4. During the last 10 minutes of roasting, heat 1 inch (2.5 cm) of water in the base of a steamer. Steam Brussels sprouts for 6 minutes, and green beans and cabbage for 3 minutes, until tender.

Nutrients per serving	
Calories	658

Total Fat
  Saturated Fat
  Omega-3
	14 g
	4 g
	0.3 g

Carbohydrate	71 g
Fiber	14 g (56% DV)
Protein	62 g
Biotin	14 mcg (5% DV)
Vitamin C	80 mg (133% DV)
Iron	5.8 mg (32% DV)
Magnesium	152 mg (38% DV)
Zinc	5 mg (33% DV)

This basic gravy is a perfect accompaniment for roasts and other meat dishes. If you are allergic to rice, use spelt flour or another eczema-safe flour (see page 78).

Eczema-Safe Gravy

1 cup	Therapeutic Broth (page 212)	250 mL
2 tsp	brown rice flour	10 mL
1 to 2 tbsp	cool filtered water	15 to 30 mL
	Garlic powder	
Pinch	sea salt, preferably Celtic (optional)	Pinch

1. In a small saucepan, bring broth to a boil over high heat. Reduce heat to a simmer.

2. In a cup, mix flour and water until lump-free. Add to the broth and simmer, stirring, until broth begins to thicken. Season to taste with garlic powder and a pinch of salt, if desired.

Health Tip

If you'd like to use salt, buy quality Celtic or natural sea salt — eczema-safe salt should be gray in color, indicating it's unprocessed and mineral-rich, and it should not contain an anti-caking agent. These alkaline salts are okay to use in moderation. Do not add salt to your food if you have high blood pressure.

Nutrients per serving	
Calories	14
Total Fat	0 g
Saturated Fat	0 g
Omega-3	0.0 g
Carbohydrate	3 g
Fiber	0 g (0% DV)
Protein	2 g
Biotin	1 mcg (0% DV)
Vitamin C	2 mg (3% DV)
Iron	1.0 mg (5% DV)
Magnesium	5 mg (1% DV)
Zinc	0 mg (0% DV)

Chicken Pasta with Green Beans

This is a basic pasta recipe that you can modify as desired. I've included instructions on how to cook it with chicken, lamb or fish.

Variation
To make this vegetarian, substitute cooked kidney beans for the chicken and skip step 2.

12 oz	boneless skinless chicken, lean lamb or eczema-safe fish (see 69), diced or sliced	375 g
1 tsp	rice bran oil	5 mL
2	cloves garlic, minced	2
8 oz	gluten-free, spelt or buckwheat pasta	250 g
½	bunch green onions, chopped	½
3	handfuls green beans, trimmed and sliced	3
½ cup	Parsley Pesto (page 241)	125 mL
5 to 6 tbsp	Therapeutic Broth (page 212) or Alkaline Veggie Broth (page 214)	75 to 90 mL
	Sea salt, preferably Celtic (optional)	

1. Place chicken in a bowl and drizzle with 1 tsp (5 mL) rice bran oil. Sprinkle with garlic and toss to coat.

2. In a wok or large nonstick skillet, over medium-high heat, stir-fry chicken until no longer pink inside (cook lamb to desired doneness; cook fish until it is opaque and flakes easily when tested with a fork). Remove from heat and cover to keep warm.

3. Meanwhile, cook pasta according to package instructions. Drain and set aside.

4. Clean skillet, then heat 1 tbsp (15 mL) water over medium heat. Lightly sauté green onions and green beans. Stir in pasta, pesto and enough broth to keep the pasta from getting dry. Season to taste with salt, if desired.

5. Divide pasta between two bowls. Top with chicken.

Nutrients per adult serving	
Calories	477

Total Fat
  Saturated Fat
  Omega-3
	16 g
	2 g
	0.1 g

Carbohydrate	55 g
Fiber	9 g (36% DV)
Protein	32 g
Biotin	21 mcg (7% DV)
Vitamin C	10 mg (17% DV)
Iron	4.4 mg (24% DV)
Magnesium	58 mg (15% DV)
Zinc	1 mg (7% DV)

My Favorite Lamb Chops

Lamb is rich in iron and vitamins A, B_2, B_3, B_5, B_6 and B_{12}. Here, it's teamed with alkalizing vegetables, including red cabbage, which supplies at least 36 different varieties of potent anthocyanins and provides antioxidant protection in the skin.

Tip

You can grill the chops if preferred.

- **Preheat oven to 450°F (230°C)**
- **Shallow baking dish, lined with parchment paper**
- **Steamer**

8	frenched lamb chops, fat trimmed (or lean lamb fillets)	8
	Rice bran oil	
	Sea salt, preferably Celtic (optional)	
3 tbsp	Parsley Pesto (page 241)	45 mL
4 to 6	large potatoes, scrubbed and chopped	4 to 6
8	Brussels sprouts, ends trimmed	8
1 cup	chopped red cabbage	250 mL
2	handfuls green beans, ends trimmed	2

1. Coat lamb cutlets in a little oil and sprinkle with salt, if desired. In a nonstick skillet, heat a splash of oil over high heat. Sear lamb for 1 minute on each side. Transfer lamb to prepared baking dish.

2. Roast lamb for 5 minutes. Turn lamb over and spread a thick layer of pesto on top. Roast for 5 minutes or until cooked to desired doneness.

3. Meanwhile, in a steamer set over a saucepan of boiling water, steam potatoes for 10 to 15 minutes, Brussels sprouts for 6 minutes, and cabbage and beans for 3 minutes, until tender.

Nutrients per serving	
Calories	550

Total Fat
    Saturated Fat
    Omega-3
	12 g
	4 g
	0.1 g

Carbohydrate	77 g
Fiber	9 g (36% DV)
Protein	33 g
Biotin	13 mcg (4% DV)
Vitamin C	121 mg (202% DV)
Iron	6.9 mg (38% DV)
Magnesium	130 mg (33% DV)
Zinc	5 mg (33% DV)

Smashed Potatoes

Makes 4 servings

Mashed potatoes with a twist — this version contains both white potatoes and sweet potato, making it rich in carotenes and vitamin C for healthy skin. Serve with grilled lamb, fish or chicken.

Tip

If you prefer, you can boil the potatoes instead of steaming them.

- **Steamer**

4 to 6	large potatoes, peeled and diced	4 to 6
1	small-medium sweet potato, peeled and diced	1
¼ cup	soy milk or rice milk	60 mL
	Sea salt, preferably Celtic	

1. In a steamer set over a saucepan of boiling water, steam potatoes and sweet potato for 10 to 15 minutes or until tender. Drain and return to the saucepan. Add milk and salt to taste. Mash to desired consistency.

Health Tip

An eczema sufferer needs to avoid many foods, so it is comforting to know you can enjoy a side of mashed potato and homemade potato wedges.

Nutrients per serving	
Calories	291

Total Fat
  Saturated Fat
  Omega-3
	1 g
	0 g
	0.0 g

Carbohydrate	67 g
Fiber	7 g (28% DV)
Protein	6 g
Biotin	4 mcg (1% DV)
Vitamin C	27 mg (45% DV)
Iron	1.2 mg (7% DV)
Magnesium	64 mg (16% DV)
Zinc	1 mg (7% DV)

Potato Wedges

Potatoes are a good source of vitamins B₃, B₆ and C and are rich in potassium. Home-baked potato wedges or chips are far healthier than packaged or restaurant versions.

Variations

Sprinkle with chopped fresh parsley before serving.

For Stage 2 only: Sprinkle with finely chopped fresh rosemary before baking.

- **Preheat oven to 400°F (200°C)**
- **Baking sheet, lined with parchment paper**

6 to 8	potatoes (with skin), scrubbed and cut into wedges	6 to 8
	Rice bran oil	
	Coarse sea salt, preferably Celtic	

1. Place potatoes in a bowl and drizzle with enough rice bran oil to lightly coat (2 tsp/10 mL or less). Toss to coat. Using a slotted spoon, transfer potatoes to prepared baking sheet and spread out in a single layer. Sprinkle with salt.

2. Bake in preheated oven for 45 to 60 minutes, turning often, until browned and crispy.

Nutrients per serving	
Calories	251
Total Fat	1 g
Saturated Fat	0 g
Omega-3	0.0 g
Carbohydrate	56 g
Fiber	7 g (28% DV)
Protein	7 g
Biotin	1 mcg (0% DV)
Vitamin C	63 mg (105% DV)
Iron	2.5 mg (14% DV)
Magnesium	74 mg (19% DV)
Zinc	1 mg (7% DV)

Chickpea Rice

<table>
<tr><td>Makes 2 servings</td></tr>
</table>

This is a fiber-rich dish with highly alkalizing mung bean sprouts and parsley. The cashews and chickpeas supply vegetarian protein. If you are not vegetarian or vegan, add Therapeutic Broth (page 212) to boost your immune system and use cooked chicken or canned tuna instead of the chickpeas, if desired.

Tip

Do not use instant brown rice.

- **Steamer**

1	small sweet potato, scrubbed	1
	Rice bran oil	
	Sea salt, preferably Celtic (optional)	
1 cup	basmati rice (or 1½ cups/375 mL brown rice)	250 mL
4 to 5	green onions, chopped	4 to 5
¼ cup	Therapeutic Broth (page 212) or Alkaline Veggie Broth (page 214)	60 mL
1 cup	cooked chickpeas (or one 14-oz/398 mL can chickpeas, drained and rinsed)	250 mL
⅓ cup	mung bean sprouts, thoroughly washed	75 mL
1	handful flat-leaf (Italian) parsley, washed and chopped	1
¼ cup	unsalted raw cashews (optional)	60 mL

1. If the skin of the sweet potato is undamaged, keep it on; otherwise, peel it. Cut sweet potato in half lengthwise, then cut into wedges.

2. In a steamer set over a saucepan of boiling water, steam sweet potato for 10 minutes or until tender.

3. Meanwhile, cook rice for 10 minutes or according to package instructions (brown rice takes about 25 minutes). Drain.

Nutrients per serving	
Calories	463

Total Fat
  Saturated Fat
  Omega-3
	5 g
	0 g
	0.0 g

Carbohydrate	97 g
Fiber	12 g (48% DV)
Protein	15 g
Biotin	35 mcg (12% DV)
Vitamin C	59 mg (98% DV)
Iron	5.5 mg (31% DV)
Magnesium	27 mg (7% DV)
Zinc	1 mg (7% DV)

Tips

Brown rice often has a high GI, so use basmati rice or a low-GI brown rice variety if you have blood sugar issues, such as diabetes. Brown rice usually takes 20 to 25 minutes to cook.

Children might prefer the green onions well cooked or fried.

4. In a nonstick skillet, lightly sauté green onions in broth. Add chickpeas and cooked rice; cook, stirring, until heated through.

5. Divide rice mixture between two shallow bowls and top with sweet potato, bean sprouts, parsley and cashews.

Variation

If you prefer, you can roast the sweet potato instead of steaming it. Coat the wedges in a little rice bran oil and sprinkle with salt, if desired. Using a slotted spoon, transfer wedges to a rimmed baking sheet lined with parchment paper and spread out in a single layer. Roast in a 400°F (200°C) oven for about 20 minutes or until tender.

Health Tip

If you are vegetarian or vegan, it is not necessary to eat red meat, fish, or chicken during the Eczema Diet. Recipes containing meat are on the menu to supply protein and iron. To meet protein and iron requirements, choose vegetarian soups and eat beans if preferred.

Quinoa

Quinoa is a nutritious gluten-free grain-like seed, perfect for those who cannot eat oats or wheat and other gluten-rich grains. Use cooked quinoa as a rice substitute or make into porridge. Favor red quinoa, as it contains powerful antioxidants called anthocyanins, which have a protective effect against UV sunlight. Serve quinoa with cooked skinless chicken, lamb, fish or beans and eczema-safe vegetables.

½ cup	red or white quinoa, rinsed	125 mL
1½ cups	filtered water	375 mL

1. In a small saucepan, combine quinoa and water. Bring to a boil, then reduce heat to low, cover and cook until quinoa is tender, about 20 minutes for white quinoa or 25 minutes for red quinoa.

Health Tip

Zinc is vital for skin repair and maintenance. Deficiency leads to skin lesions, dry and rough skin, and delayed wound healing.

Nutrients per serving	
Calories	313

Total Fat
  Saturated Fat
  Omega-3
	5 g
	1 g
	0.3 g

Carbohydrate	55 g
Fiber	6 g (24% DV)
Protein	12 g
Biotin	0 mcg (0% DV)
Vitamin C	0 mg (0% DV)
Iron	3.9 mg (22% DV)
Magnesium	171 mg (43% DV)
Zinc	3 mg (20% DV)

Snacks and Sweets

Banana Carob Spread

Makes ½ cup (125 mL)

This alkalizing spread is rich in fiber and potassium. Use it on Spelt Lavash Bread (page 243), toast, pancakes, rice crackers or fruit salad.

Tip

If a smooth paste is desired, blend in a small food processor.

1	ripe medium banana, mashed	1
1 tsp	carob powder	5 mL
1 tsp	rice malt syrup (optional)	5 mL
	Ascorbic acid or citric acid (optional)	

1. In a bowl, combine banana and carob. Taste and, if desired, stir in rice malt syrup (for added sweetness) and a sprinkle of ascorbic acid (for tang).

2. Store in an airtight container in the refrigerator for up to 2 days.

Health Tip

Ideally, your diet should have no added sweeteners, but for those of you who wish to use sweeteners, the best choice is rice malt syrup, for two reasons: it is alkalizing, whereas all other sweeteners convert to acid in the body, and it is low in salicylates and other chemicals. Rice malt syrup is milder than honey, so more may be required in recipes.

Nutrients per 1 tbsp (15 mL)	
Calories	14
Total Fat Saturated Fat Omega-3	0 g 0 g 0.0 g
Carbohydrate	4 g
Fiber	0 g (0% DV)
Protein	0 g
Biotin	0 mcg (0% DV)
Vitamin C	0 mg (0% DV)
Iron	0.1 mg (1% DV)
Magnesium	4 mg (1% DV)
Zinc	0 mg (0% DV)

Sesame-Free Hummus

Makes 2¼ cups (550 mL)

Serve this delicious hummus with crackers and veggie sticks, add a dollop to salads or spread it on sandwiches or toast for a protein-rich snack, breakfast or lunch.

Tips

This dip is wonderfully garlicky. You may want to reduce the garlic used initially and add more after sampling.

If you are breastfeeding, or if your baby is gassy or has colic, you may need to avoid using raw garlic and green onions.

If making this for a child, you may wish to skip the garlic and ascorbic acid and reduce the green onions.

Nutrients per ¼ cup (60 mL)	
Calories	52

Total Fat
  Saturated Fat
  Omega-3
	2 g
	0 g
	0.0 g

Carbohydrate	7 g
Fiber	2 g (8% DV)
Protein	2 g
Biotin	10 mcg (3% DV)
Vitamin C	1 mg (2% DV)
Iron	0.5 mg (3% DV)
Magnesium	0 mg (0% DV)
Zinc	0 mg (0% DV)

- **Food processor**

1½ cups	cooked chickpeas (or one 14 oz/398 mL can chickpeas, drained and rinsed)	375 mL
1	small clove garlic, minced	1
1 tbsp	rice bran oil	15 mL
6 tbsp	filtered water	90 mL
¼ tsp	ascorbic acid or citric acid (optional)	1 mL
¼ tsp	sea salt, preferably Celtic	1 mL
¼ cup	chopped green onions, green parts only	60 mL

1. In food processor, combine chickpeas, garlic, rice bran oil, 5 tbsp (75 mL) water, ascorbic acid (if desired for tang), salt and green onions; process until smooth. Taste and adjust if necessary. Add more water if a thinner consistency is desired.

2. Store in an airtight container in the refrigerator for up to 3 days.

Bean Dip

**Makes 2 cups
(500 mL)**

Beans are a good source of vegetarian protein, and this eczema-safe dip can be used to flavor your salads or to accompany rice crackers.

- **Blender**

1½ cups	cooked kidney beans (or one 14-oz/398 mL can red kidney beans, drained and rinsed)	375 mL
1	small clove garlic	1
1 tbsp	rice bran oil	15 mL
¼ tsp	citric acid	1 mL
⅓ cup	filtered water (approx.)	75 mL

1. In blender, combine beans, garlic, rice bran oil, citric acid and water; blend until smooth, adding more water if necessary.

2. Store in an airtight container in the refrigerator for up to 3 days.

Health Tip

Legumes are rich in magnesium and potassium and supply dietary fiber, protein, and slow-release carbohydrates for energy. If using canned legumes, it is essential to drain and thoroughly rinse them because they are packed with a fair amount of salt. Dried legumes that are home-cooked are the best and most nutritious choice.

Nutrients per ¼ cup (60 mL)	
Calories	62

Total Fat
  Saturated Fat
  Omega-3
	2 g
	0 g
	0.0 g

Carbohydrate	9 g
Fiber	3 g (12% DV)
Protein	3 g
Biotin	2 mcg (1% DV)
Vitamin C	0 mg (0% DV)
Iron	0.8 mg (4% DV)
Magnesium	0 mg (0% DV)
Zinc	0 mg (0% DV)

Parsley Pesto

<table>
<tr><td colspan="2">**Makes 1¾ cups (425 mL)**</td></tr>
</table>

This delicious protein-rich, alkalizing spread is perfect for special occasions. Spread it on plain rice crackers, whole-grain rye crispbread, sourdough toast and sandwiches, or add it to gluten-free or spelt pasta for a quick meal. Parsley Pesto is not suitable if you have a nut allergy of any kind. Large amounts of parsley contain salicylates, so eat only in moderation.

Tip

Use the ascorbic acid or citric acid if you prefer a tangy flavor. Citric acid is usually found in the baking section of large supermarkets or in pharmacies.

Nutrients per ¼ cup (60 mL)	
Calories	179
Total Fat	16 g
Saturated Fat	3 g
Omega-3	0.1 g
Carbohydrate	6 g
Fiber	1 g (4% DV)
Protein	4 g
Biotin	5 mcg (2% DV)
Vitamin C	6 mg (10% DV)
Iron	1.6 mg (9% DV)
Magnesium	60 mg (15% DV)
Zinc	1 mg (7% DV)

- **Food processor**

1	large bunch parsley	1
¼ cup	rice bran oil	60 mL
1 cup	unsalted raw cashews	250 mL
¼ cup	filtered water	60 mL
1 tsp	minced garlic, or to taste	5 mL
¼ tsp	ascorbic acid or citric acid (optional)	1 mL
¼ tsp	sea salt, preferably Celtic (optional)	1 mL

1. Trim half the stems off the parsley, wash the leaves in a bowl of water and shake off any excess water.

2. In food processor, combine parsley, rice bran oil, cashews, water, garlic, ascorbic acid (if using) and salt (if using); process until smooth. Taste and add more garlic or seasoning, if desired.

3. Store in an airtight container in the refrigerator for up to 3 days.

Variation

Beet and Cashew Dip: Boil 1 medium beet for 30 minutes or until soft, then peel and chop. Skip step 1 and replace the parsley with the beet.

Baked Banana Chips

Makes 4 servings

These alkalizing and additive-free banana chips are naturally sweet treats that are chewy rather than crispy. You'll just need a bit of time and a pastry brush. If you have a dehydrator, you can use it instead of baking.

Variation

If you are sensitive to lemon juice, brush banana slices with a little rice bran oil instead of lemon juice.

- **Preheat oven to 200°F (100°C)**
- **Baking sheet, lined with parchment paper**

| 2 | ripe large bananas | 2 |
| 1/2 | lemon, juiced | 1/2 |

1. Slice the bananas a little less than $1/4$ inch (0.5 cm) thick and on the diagonal (they shrink a lot, so don't cut them too thin). Arrange on prepared baking sheet and brush each one on both sides with a little lemon juice.

2. Bake in preheated oven for 2 to 3 hours, turning every 30 minutes, until bananas are dehydrated (remove before excessive browning).

3. Store in an airtight container at room temperature for up to 1 week.

Nutrients per serving	
Calories	54

Total Fat
  Saturated Fat
  Omega-3
	0 g
	0 g
	0.0 g

Carbohydrate	14 g
Fiber	2 g (8% DV)
Protein	1 g
Biotin	2 mcg (1% DV)
Vitamin C	8 mg (13% DV)
Iron	0.2 mg (1% DV)
Magnesium	16 mg (4% DV)
Zinc	0 mg (0% DV)

Spelt Lavash Bread

Makes 6 flatbreads

This flatbread is delicious and easy to make. For topping suggestions, see Design Your Own Sandwich (page 223).

Tip

For soft wraps, cook them quickly.

Variation

Spelt Chips: Roll out each ball of dough until very thin. Cut out triangles and place on baking sheets lined with parchment paper. Bake in a preheated 350°F (180°C) oven for 10 minutes or until crisp.

1¼ cups	spelt flour, preferably whole-grain	300 mL
¾ tsp	fine sea salt, preferably Celtic	3 mL
1 tbsp	rice bran oil	15 mL
⅔ cup	boiling water	150 mL
	Spelt flour	

1. In a bowl, combine spelt flour and salt. Using a knife, stir in rice bran oil and boiling water. The dough should be soft but not sticky. (Depending on the brand of flour you use, you may need more hot water. Add it 1 tsp/5 mL at a time.)

2. On a lightly floured cutting board, knead dough for about 3 minutes, until smooth and elastic. Cut into 6 pieces and form into balls.

3. On a floured board, roll out each ball into a large, thin circle (the thinner, the better).

4. Heat a large nonstick skillet over high heat. Cook each flatbread for 1 minute per side, or until bubbles appear. Gently pop the bubbles before they burn. Reduce heat if necessary to avoid burning.

Health Tip

When testing wheat, choose quality wheat products first, such as whole wheat sourdough bread. If an adverse reaction occurs, note it in your diet diary, discontinue use, and re-test the food in 1 to 2 months' time if desired.

Nutrients per flatbread	
Calories	112

Total Fat
  Saturated Fat
  Omega-3
	3 g
	1 g
	0.0 g

Carbohydrate	19 g
Fiber	2 g (8% DV)
Protein	4 g
Biotin	2 mcg (1% DV)
Vitamin C	0 mg (0% DV)
Iron	0.9 mg (5% DV)
Magnesium	0 mg (0% DV)
Zinc	0 mg (0% DV)

Roasted Potato Snack

Makes 2 servings

This nutritious lunch is rich in alkalizing vegetables and balanced with protein. If you are vegetarian or vegan, omit the fish.

Variation

Replace the beet dip with another eczema-safe dip.

- **Preheat oven to 400°F (200°C)**
- **Rimmed baking sheet, lined with parchment paper**

3	large potatoes (or 1 small sweet potato), scrubbed	3
½ tsp	rice bran oil	2 mL
1 cup	romaine lettuce	250 mL
1	can (3 oz/85 g) drained water-packed canned tuna or other eczema-safe fish	1
3 tbsp	Beet and Cashew Dip (variation, page 241)	45 mL
¼ cup	mung bean sprouts, thoroughly washed	60 mL

1. Cut potatoes in half lengthwise and place on prepared baking sheet. Brush with a little rice bran oil. Roast in preheated oven for 30 minutes or until tender.

2. Serve potatoes beside the lettuce and top potatoes with tuna, dip and bean sprouts.

Nutrients per serving	
Calories	387

Total Fat
    Saturated Fat
    Omega-3
	9 g
	2 g
	0.5 g

Carbohydrate	60 g
Fiber	8 g (32% DV)
Protein	19 g
Biotin	3 mcg (1% DV)
Vitamin C	70 mg (117% DV)
Iron	3.7 mg (21% DV)
Magnesium	113 mg (28% DV)
Zinc	2 mg (13% DV)

The Wishing Plate

Makes 2 servings

Serve these eczema-safe veggies each afternoon to help meet your or your child's alkalizing veggie quota for the day. Serve with Sesame-Free Hummus (page 239) or another eczema-safe dip, if desired.

Tip

Use the Wishing Plate as a healthy and fun way to "market" veggies to your child. Buy a decorative plate to use exclusively as the Wishing Plate (like it is a sacred ritual). Tell them, "Each time you eat a veggie from the Wishing Plate, you get to make a wish."

1	carrot, peeled and cut into sticks and/or circles	1
1	stalk celery, strings peeled, cut into sticks or "shark's teeth"	1
1 tbsp	mung bean sprouts (remove green shells, if desired) or sprouted lentils (see page 66)	15 mL

1. Arrange vegetables on a fun-looking plate if serving to children. Young children may want their veggies arranged into shapes (clock, truck, flower and so on), or they can create their own arrangement. After eating a veggie (or sprout), make a wish.

Health Tip

According to some recent research, Americans continue to suffer from scurvy (the "sailor's disease" of the 1700s) because people aren't eating enough fruit and vegetables.

Nutrients per serving	
Calories	19

Total Fat
  Saturated Fat
  Omega-3
	0 g
	0 g
	0.0 g

Carbohydrate	4 g
Fiber	1 g (4% DV)
Protein	1 g
Biotin	2 mcg (1% DV)
Vitamin C	5 mg (8% DV)
Iron	0.2 mg (1% DV)
Magnesium	4 mg (1% DV)
Zinc	0 mg (0% DV)

Eczema-Safe Fruit Salad

Makes 2 servings

Papaya is rich in vitamin C and lycopene, which, if consumed frequently, works as a protective sunscreen in the skin. It's teamed with fiber- and potassium-rich banana and pear. Flax seeds are rich in omega-3s, and lecithin supplies choline and inositol for healthy skin cell membranes.

Tip

If you're allergic or sensitive to soy, omit the soy lecithin granules.

1	pear, peeled and diced	1
1	ripe banana, chopped	1
2	slices papaya, diced	2
2 tsp	whole flax seeds, soaked overnight if desired	10 mL
2 tsp	soy lecithin granules	10 mL

1. In a bowl, combine pear, banana, papaya, flax seeds and soy lecithin.

Health Tip

After antibiotic use or a bout of illness, you can eat a serving of papaya daily to promote recolonization of beneficial bacteria in the gastrointestinal tract.

Nutrients per serving	
Calories	193
Total Fat 　Saturated Fat 　Omega-3	3 g 1 g 0.8 g
Carbohydrate	42 g
Fiber	7 g (28% DV)
Protein	2 g
Biotin	2 mcg (1% DV)
Vitamin C	55 mg (92% DV)
Iron	0.9 mg (5% DV)
Magnesium	38 mg (10% DV)
Zinc	1 mg (7% DV)

Stewed Pears

Makes 4 servings	4	large pears, peeled and sliced into thick wedges	4
		Filtered water

Peeled pears are very low in salicylates, and stewed pears make a simple and healthy dessert. Mashed stewed pears are also ideal for infants with eczema (see tip, below).

1. Place pears and water in a saucepan. Bring to a boil over high heat and boil for 3 minutes or until tender (if making for dessert, don't cook for too long or the pears will go mushy). Remove from heat and strain off the liquid (you can keep this for drinking).

Tips

For baby food, dice the pears and steam them until they start to go mushy (about 15 minutes), then mash the pears with a fork. You can freeze leftovers in an ice cube tray, cover and defrost some each day.

You can use puréed stewed pear to make icy poles (see page 251) for your child.

Variation

For Stage 2 only: Make stewed apples and add a sprinkling of blueberries (both contain salicylates).

Nutrients per serving	
Calories	133

Total Fat
  Saturated Fat
  Omega-3
	0 g
	0 g
	0.0 g

Carbohydrate	36 g
Fiber	7 g (28% DV)
Protein	1 g
Biotin	1 mcg (0% DV)
Vitamin C	10 mg (17% DV)
Iron	0.4 mg (2% DV)
Magnesium	16 mg (4% DV)
Zinc	0 mg (0% DV)

Birthday Cake

Makes 10 servings

This dairy-free, gluten-free vanilla cake is perfect for people who are sensitive to dairy and gluten. Preferably use a cake pan that has a hole in the middle. Give your cake the wow factor by using a fluted cake pan. You can also use this recipe to make gluten-free cupcakes (medium-size cupcakes bake in about 10 minutes).

Tip
Buckwheat flour is incredibly nutritious and rich in quercetin, and it can help counteract some of the inflammatory effects of the refined sugar.

- **Preheat oven to 350°F (180°C)**
- **Food processor**
- **9-inch (23 cm) fluted or round cake pan, oiled with rice bran oil**

2¼ cups	all-purpose gluten-free flour mix	550 mL
2 tbsp	buckwheat flour (optional)	30 mL
1 cup	fine raw sugar	250 mL
4 tsp	baking powder	20 mL
¼ tsp	fine sea salt (see tip, at right)	1 mL
2	large eggs (or equivalent egg substitute)	2
1 cup	rice milk	250 mL
½ tsp	vanilla extract	2 mL
⅓ cup	rice bran oil	75 mL

1. In a large bowl, combine flour mix, buckwheat flour, sugar, baking powder and salt.

2. In food processor, combine eggs, rice milk and vanilla; process until well combined. With the motor running, slowly drizzle oil through the chute; process until smooth and creamy.

3. Pour liquid over flour mixture and stir in with a wooden spoon. Spread in prepared cake pan.

Nutrients per serving	
Calories	251

Total Fat
  Saturated Fat
  Omega-3
	9 g
	2 g
	0.1 g

Carbohydrate	42 g
Fiber	3 g (12% DV)
Protein	4 g
Biotin	5 mcg (2% DV)
Vitamin C	0 mg (0% DV)
Iron	1.2 mg (7% DV)
Magnesium	2 mg (1% DV)
Zinc	0 mg (0% DV)

Tips

Check your gluten-free flour mix to see if there is salt in the ingredients. If there is, omit the added salt in this recipe.

If your gluten-free flour mix contains guar gum, you may need an extra $\frac{1}{4}$ cup (60 mL) rice milk ($1\frac{1}{4}$ cups/300 mL total).

If you cannot find rice bran oil, use refined (high heat) safflower oil, with no added antioxidants.

Store at room temperature for up to 24 hours (cakes are softer if not refrigerated before the party). Store leftovers in an airtight container in the refrigerator.

To ice this cake, use gluten-free confectioners' (icing) sugar mixed with a little water, and drizzle or spread it on. Or dust the top of the cake with gluten-free confectioners' (icing) sugar.

4. Bake in preheated oven for 20 to 30 minutes or until a tester inserted in the center comes out clean (if the pan has a hole in the center, the baking time will be closer to 20 minutes). Let cool for 5 minutes before removing cake from the pan.

Health Tip

Gluten intolerance can restrict the grains your child can eat and make it difficult to meet nutrient requirements. If your child cannot eat gluten, you will be able to convert most recipes into gluten-free versions by substituting other grains.

New Anzac Cookies

Makes 20 cookies

These sweet cookies are egg- and dairy-free, rich in dietary fiber and suitable for snacks, parties and lunch box treats. Although this recipe is wheat-free, it's not suitable if you have a wheat allergy or gluten intolerance, as spelt contains gluten and oats may contain traces of wheat.

- **Preheat oven to 300°F (150°C)**
- **Baking sheets, lined with parchment paper**

1½ cups	rolled oats	375 mL
1 cup	spelt flour, preferably whole-grain	250 mL
⅔ cup	fine raw sugar	150 mL
½ cup	rice bran oil	125 mL
1 tbsp	maple syrup	15 mL
1½ tsp	baking soda	7 mL
1 to 3 tbsp	water	15 to 45 mL

1. In a bowl, combine oats, spelt flour and sugar.

2. In a small saucepan, over high heat, combine rice bran oil and syrup. Cook, stirring constantly, until syrup begins to bubble. Immediately add baking soda, stirring until it foams. Quickly remove from heat and pour the hot foaming liquid onto the dry ingredients and mix well. Stir in water, 1 tbsp (15 mL) at a time, until the dough sticks together.

3. Form dough into 20 small balls (about ¾ inch/2 cm wide) and place on prepared baking sheets (they will expand, so allow room between them).

4. Bake in preheated oven for 12 to 15 minutes or until golden brown.

Nutrients per cookie	
Calories	103

Total Fat
    Saturated Fat
    Omega-3
	6 g
	1 g
	0.1 g

Carbohydrate	13 g
Fiber	1 g (4% DV)
Protein	1 g
Biotin	2 mcg (1% DV)
Vitamin C	0 mg (0% DV)
Iron	0.3 mg (2% DV)
Magnesium	0 mg (0% DV)
Zinc	0 mg (0% DV)

Banana Icy Poles

Makes 4 servings

These healthy, alkalizing icy poles can be enjoyed daily or for occasional treats. Lecithin supplies choline and inositol for healthy skin cell membranes, but you can omit it if you are allergic to soy.

Variation

Use soy milk instead of rice milk and add vanilla extract or a sprinkle of carob powder.

- **Blender**
- **Plastic ice pop mold**

1	large ripe banana, mashed	1
1 tsp	soy lecithin granules (optional)	5 mL
1 tsp	rice malt syrup	5 mL
½ cup	rice milk	125 mL

1. In a blender, combine banana, lecithin (if using), rice malt syrup and rice milk; blend until smooth.

2. Transfer mixture to ice pop mold and freeze until hard (it's best to let them set overnight).

Health Tip

In order of preference, here are the sweeteners eczema sufferers can use in recipes:

- Rice malt syrup (alkalizing, low in chemicals)
- Pure maple syrup (acid-producing, low in chemicals)
- Golden syrup (acid-producing, low in chemicals)

Nutrients per serving	
Calories	55

Total Fat
  Saturated Fat
  Omega-3
	0 g
	0 g
	0.0 g

Carbohydrate	13 g
Fiber	1 g (4% DV)
Protein	1 g
Biotin	1 mcg (0% DV)
Vitamin C	3 mg (5% DV)
Iron	0.1 mg (1% DV)
Magnesium	12 mg (3% DV)
Zinc	0 mg (0% DV)

Bananas on Sticks

Makes 2 servings

Bananas are alkalizing and, when frozen, have the consistency of ice cream. They make a healthy dessert or guilt-free snack for when you are craving something sweet.

- **2 ice pop sticks**
- 2   small ripe bananas, peeled   2

1. Put the bananas on ice pop sticks by piercing them through one end. Wrap each banana in plastic wrap. Freeze overnight. They will last up to 1 week in the freezer.

Health Tip

Bananas are a fiber-rich and nutritious energy snack. Although they contain some amines, they also supply their own amine- and histamine-lowering nutrients, magnesium and vitamin C, so this nutrient-dense snack should not pose a problem for those who are mildly sensitive to amines.

Nutrients per serving	
Calories	105

Total Fat
  Saturated Fat
  Omega-3
	0 g
	0 g
	0.3 g

Carbohydrate	27 g
Fiber	3 g (12% DV)
Protein	1 g
Biotin	3 mcg (1% DV)
Vitamin C	10 mg (17% DV)
Iron	0.3 mg (2% DV)
Magnesium	32 mg (8% DV)
Zinc	0 mg (0% DV)

Acknowledgments

I have many people to thank for their input during the creation of the Eczema Diet. Firstly, my daughter was the inspiration for this research and she helped design two of the dessert recipes. My children, Ayva and Jack, are the first people to test my recipes and they have helped me to grow in so many ways, so I dedicate this book to both of them.

Over the years, my patients and readers have inspired me to continue researching eczema. In particular, a boy called Jacob whose mother wrote to me months after their initial consultation to tell me of the pain and embarrassment Jacob had suffered while he had eczema and how happy they both felt when Jacob's skin healed. The before and after photos of Jacob brought tears to my eyes and I resolved to continue with my work. I really appreciate the feedback from my former patients and I admire their dedication to follow the diet and improve their skin (and on occasion, tell me straight what's working and what isn't!). Thank you all for your feedback, especially Mary Washington, Amanda Essex, Linda Balfour, Natalya L., Bianca Rothwell, Anandhi Krishnakumar, Claudine Hardy, Meaghan Ottewill, Karma Montagne, Bronwyn Air, Jenny Bangor, Lyn McPherson, Cathi Firth, and Anna Kluge. And thanks to Bianca Rothwell for forwarding a couple of her recipes so I could pass them on to other eczema sufferers.

My mother is my greatest support and I owe her a mountain of gratitude for her advice, love, and encouragement, and my dad, for his interest in health — both of you have provided me with a strong foundation to persevere in my field of work, which I adore.

I really appreciate the words of support from Professor Gary Leong, director of KOALA Healthy Life Clinic at the Mater Children's Hospital — thank you for your testimonials and encouragement over the past 3 years.

I want to thank Professor Michael J. Cork, Head of Academic Unit of Dermatology Research, and Les Hunter from the University of Sheffield, who kindly supplied the "brick wall model of the skin" illustration. The liver detoxification data obtained from HealthScope Pathology in Melbourne, and the scientific research on eczema, allergies, nutrients, and food intolerance, were instrumental in creating and refining this program, so I'd like to thank all scientists and medical researchers for publishing their valuable work. The Eczema Association of Australasia does a wonderful job supporting eczema sufferers and I'm grateful for their newsletters, support, and online information.

I'd like to say a heartfelt thank you to Selwa Anthony for believing in my writing and to Benny St John Thomas and the team at Exisle Publishing for publishing my books and for making them look beautiful. A special thank you goes to my editors Anouska Jones and Karen Gee: I feel so blessed to have editors who understand health and they enhance my work in so many ways.

This has been a long process and I'm sure my eczema research will continue.

I wish I could have supplied more recipes in this book, but the present ones took me 10 years to design and refine. To increase variety, I encourage you to experiment with the eczema-safe ingredients and design additional recipes for yourself, and if you'd like to see your eczema-safe recipes (and your name) in the next book, you can submit your recipes for review via my website. Thank you for reading my books and for entrusting me with your health. May your eczema heal swiftly.

Warm wishes,
Karin

Resources

● ●

Health Before Beauty
(my free health information website)
For skin-care and product reviews, log on to www.healthbeforebeauty.com

Fischer, Karen. *The 8-Week Healthy Skin Diet*. Toronto: Robert Rose, 2013.

Fischer, Karen. *Healthy Family, Happy Family*. Australia and New Zealand: Exisle Publishing, 2011.

References

Anderson, R.A., et al., 1991, Supplemental-chromium effects on glucose, insulin, glucagon, and urinary chromium losses in subjects consuming controlled low-chromium diets, *American Journal of Clinical Nutrition*, vol. 54, pp. 909–16.

Baugh, C.M., Malone, J.H., and Butterworth, C.E., 1968, Human biotin deficiency, *American Journal of Clinical Nutrition*, vol. 21, pp. 173–182.

Beare, J.M., 1968, The association between candida albicans and lesions of seborrhoeic eczema, *British Journal of Dermatology*, vol. 80, no. 10, pp. 675–81.

Boelsma, E., et al., 2003, Human skin condition and its associations with nutrient concentrations in serum and diet, *American Journal of Clinical Nutrition*, vol. 77, pp. 348–55.

Bolte, G., et al., 2001, Margarine consumption and allergy in children, *American Journal of Respiratory and Critical Care Medicine*, vol. 163, pp. 277–79.

Booken, D., et al., 2008, Glycine receptors are present in human epidermis, *Open Journal of Dermatology*, vol. 2, pp 51–56.

Brenninkmeijer, E.E.A., et al., 2008, Diagnostic criteria for atopic dermatitis: a systematic review, *British Journal of Dermatology*, vol. 158, pp. 754–65.

Caffarelli, C., et al., 1998, Gastrointestinal symptoms in atopic eczema, *Archives of Disease in Childhood*, vol. 78, pp. 230–34.

Clemetson, C.A.B., 2003, Elevated blood histamine caused by vaccinations and vitamin C deficiency may mimic the shaken baby syndrome, *Medical Hypothesis*, vol. 62, no. 4, pp. 533–36.

Cordain, L. et al., 2002, Acne vulgaris, a disease of Western civilisation, *Archives of Dermatology*, vol. 138, no. 12, pp. 1584–90.

Cordain, L., et al., 2005, Origins and evolution of the Western diet: health implications for the 21st century, *American Journal of Clinical Nutrition*, vol. 81, pp. 341–54.

Cordain. L., 2005, Implications for the role of diet in acne, Seminars in Cutaneous Medicine and Surgery, vol. 24, no. 2, reprinted in *Rosacea News*, Could rosacea be caused by diet?

Cork, M.J., et al., New understanding to the predisposition of atopic eczema and sensitive skin, retrieved 1 May 2011: www.allergyuk.org

Cork, M.J., et al., 2006, New perspectives on epidermal barrier dysfunction in atopic dermatitis: gene-environment interactions, *Journal of Allergy and Clinical Immunology*, vol. 118, pp. 3–21.

Dawson, T.L., 2007, Malassezia globosa and restricta: breakthrough understanding of the etiology and treatment of dandruff and seborrheic dermatitis through whole-genome analysis, *Journal of Investigative Dermatology Symposium Proceedings*, vol. 12, pp. 15–9.

De Spirt, S., et al., 2009, Intervention with flaxseed and borage oil supplements modulates skin condition in women, *British Journal of Nutrition*, vol. 101, pp. 440–45.

DeMeo, M.T., et al., 2002, Intestinal permeation and gastrointestinal disease, *Journal of Clinical Gastroenterology*, vol. 34, no. 4, pp. 385–96.

Dengate, S., Annato (160b), Food Intolerance Network fact sheet: http://www.fedupwith foodadditives.info/factsheets/Factannatto.htm

Dengate, S., 2009, Sulphites (220–228), Food Intolerance Network fact sheet: http://www.fedupwithfoodadditives.info/ factsheets/ Factsulphites.htm

Do, R., et al., 2011, The effect of chromosome 9p21 variants on cardiovascular disease may be modified by dietary intake: evidence from a case/control and a prospective study, *PLoS Medicine*, vol. 9, no. 10, retrieved 20 October 2011: www.plosmedicine.org

Ehrlich, S.D., 2009, Alpha-lipoic acid, University of Maryland Medical Centre website, retrieved 1 September 2011: www.umm.edu/altmed/articles/alpha-lipoic-000285.htm

Ehrlich, S.D., 2009, Calcium, University of Maryland Medical Center, retrieved 7 September 2011: www.umm.edu/altmed/articles/calcium-000290.htm

Ehrlich, S.D., 2009, Quercetin, University of Maryland Medical Center website, retrieved 1 September 2011: http://www.umm.edu/altmed/ articles/quercetin-000322.htm

Fiddler, W., et al., 1978, Inhibition of formation of volatile nitrosamines in fried bacon by the use of cure-solubilized α-tocopherol, *Journal of Agriculture and Food Chemistry*, vol. 26, no. 3, pp. 653–56.

Fiddler, W., et al., 1998, Nitrosamine formation in processed hams as related to reformulated elastic rubber netting, *Journal of Food Science*, vol. 63, pp. 276–78.

Frassetto, L.A., et al., 1998, Estimation of net endogenous noncarbonic acid production in humans from diet potassium and protein contents, *American Journal of Clinical Nutrition*, vol. 68, pp. 576–83.

Galli, E., et al., 1994, Analysis of polyunsaturated fatty acids in newborn sera: a screening tool for atopic disease? *British Journal of Dermatology*, vol. 130, pp. 752–56.

Garc Roché, M.O., 2006, Effect of ascorbic acid on the hepatotoxicity due to the daily intake of nitrate, nitrite and dimethylamine, *Food/Nahrung*, vol. 31, no. 2, pp. 99–104.

Gundersen, R.Y., et al., 2005, Glycine — an important neurotransmitter and cytoprotective agent, *Acta Anaesthesiologica Scandinavica*, vol. 49. no. 8, pp. 1108–16.

Gupta, C., et al., 2010, Antioxidant and antimutagenic effect of quercetin against DEN induced hepatotoxicity in rats, *Phytotherapy Research*, vol. 24, no. 1, pp. 119–28.

Gutman, A.B., Yu, T.F., and Sirota, J.H., 1955, A study by simultaneous clearance techniques of salicylate excretion in man. Effect of alkalinization of the urine by bicarbonate administration; effect of probenecid, *Journal of Clinical Investigation*, vol. 34, no. 5, pp. 711–21.

Hawrelak, J., 2002, Probiotics: are supplements really better than yogurt? *Journal of the Australian Traditional-Medicine Society*, vol. 8, no. 1, pp. 11–23.

Hawrelak, J., 2003, Probiotics: choosing the right one for your needs, *Journal of the Australian Traditional-Medicine Society*, vol. 9, no. 2, pp. 67–75.

Heinrich, J., et al., 2001, Allergic sensitization and diet: ecological analysis in selected European cities, *European Respiratory Journal*, vol. 17, no. 3, pp. 395–402.

Hix, L., et al., 2004, Bioactive carotenoids: potent antioxidants and regulators of gene expression, *Redox Report*, vol. 9, no. 4, pp. 181–91.

Holick, M.F., 2007, Vitamin D deficiency, *New England Journal of Medicine*, vol. 357, no. 3, pp. 266–81.

Honikel, K.O., 2008, The use and control of nitrate and nitrite for the processing of meat products, Meat Science, retrieved 16 April 2011: www.sciencedirect.com

Horrobin, D.F., 2000, Essential fatty acid metabolism and its modification in atopic eczema, *American Journal of Clinical Nutrition*, vol. 71, no. 1, pp. S367–72.

Ionescu, G.J., 2009, New insights in the pathogenesis of atopic disease, *Journal of Medicine and Life*, vol. 2, no. 2, pp. 145–54.

Isolauri E., et al., 2000, Probiotics in the management of atopic eczema, *Clinical and Experimental Allergy*, vol. 30, pp. 1604–10.

Jackson, P.G., et al., 1981, Intestinal permeability in patients with eczema and food allergy, *The Lancet*, vol. 1, no. 8233, pp. 1285–86.

Jerome, J.J., et al. 1976, Inhibition of amine-nitrite hepatotoxicity by α-tocopherol, *Toxicology and Applied Pharmacology*, vol. 41, no. 3, pp. 575–83.

Johnston, C.S., et al., 1992, Antihistamine effect of supplemental ascorbic acid and neutrophil chemotaxis, *Journal of the American College of Nutrition*, vol. 11, no. 2, pp. 172–76.

Johnston, C.S., et al., 1996, Vitamin C depletion is associated with alterations in blood histamine and plasma free carnitine in adults, *Journal of the American College of Nutrition*, vol. 15, pp. 586–91.

Kahraman, A., et al., 2003, The antioxidative and antihistaminic properties of quercetin in ethanol-induced gastric lesions, *Toxicology*, vol. 183, no. 1–3, pp. 133–42.

Kalliomäki, M., et al., 2001, Probiotics in primary prevention of atopic disease: a randomised placebo-controlled trial, *The Lancet*, vol. 357, pp. 1076–9.

Kalliomäki M., et al., 2003, Probiotics and prevention of atopic disease: 4-year follow-up of a randomised placebo-controlled trial, *The Lancet*, vol. 361, no. 9372, pp. 1869–71.

Kelble, A., 2005, Spices and type 2 diabetes, *Nutrition and Food Science*, vol. 35, no. 2, pp. 81–7.

Kimata, H., 2007, Laughter elevates the levels of breastmilk melatonin, *Journal of Psychosomatic Research*, vol. 62, no. 6, pp. 699–702.

Kurtz, I., et al., 1983, Effect of diet on plasma acid-base composition in normal humans, *Kidney International*, vol. 24, pp. 670–80.

Liska, D. J., 1998, The detoxification enzyme systems, *Alternative Medicine Review*, vol. 3, no. 3, pp. 187–98.

Loblay, R.H. and Swain, A.R., 2006, Food intolerance, *Recent Advances in Clinical Nutrition*, University of Sydney, RPA Hospital.

Loblay, R.H. and Swain, A.R., 2006, Food Intolerance, *Recent Advances in Clinical Nutrition*, retrieved 1 April 2011: www.nsw.gov.au.

Ly, N.P., et al., 2011, Gut microbiota, probiotics and vitamin D: interrelated exposures influencing allergy, asthma and obesity, *Clinical Reviews in Allergy and Immunology*, vol. 127, pp. 1087–94.

Maintz, L. and Novak, N., 2007, Histamine and histamine intolerance, *American Journal of Clinical Nutrition*, vol. 85, no. 5, pp. 1185–96.

Maintz, L., et al., 2006, Evidence for a reduced histamine degradation capacity in a subgroup of patients with atopic eczema, *Journal of Allergy and Clinical Immunology*, vol. 117, no. 5, pp. 1106–12.

Manku, M.S., 1984, Essential fatty acids in the plasma phospholipids of patients with atopic eczema, *British Journal of Dermatology*, vol. 110, pp. 643–48.

Manz, F., 2001, History of nutrition and acid-base physiology, *European Journal of Nutrition*, vol. 40, pp. 189–99.

McCann, D., et al., 2007, Food additives and hyperactive behaviour in 3-year-old and 8/9-year-old children in the community: a randomised, double-blinded, placebo-controlled trial, *The Lancet*, vol. 370, pp. 1560–67.

McGinley, K.J., et al., 1975, Quantitative microbiology of the scalp in non-dandruff and seborrheic dermatitis, *Journal of Investigative Dermatology*, vol. 64, no. 6, pp. 401–05.

Meydani, S.N., et al., 1991, Vitamin B6 deficiency impairs interleukin 2 production and lymphocyte proliferation in elderly adults, *American Journal of Clinical Nutrition*, vol. 53, no. 5, pp. 1275–80.

Mine, Y. and Yang, M., 2008, Recent advances in the understanding of egg allergens: basic, industrial, and clinical perspectives, *Journal of Agricultural and Food Chemistry*, vol. 56, pp. 4874–900.

Minich, D.M. and Bland, J.S., 2007, Acid–alkaline balance: role in chronic disease and detoxification, *Alternative Therapies*, vol. 13, no. 4, pp. 62–65.

Nakanishi, Y., et al, 2008, Monosodium glutamate (MSG): a villain and promoter of liver inflammation and dysplasia, *Journal of Autoimmunity*, vol. 30, no. 1–2, pp. 42–50.

New, S.A., 2001, Fruit and vegetable consumption and skeletal health: is there a positive link? *Nutrition Bulletin*, vol. 26, no. 2, pp. 121–25.

O'Malley, G.F., 2007, Emergency department management of the salicylate-poisoned patient, *Emergency Medicine Clinics of North America*, vol. 25, pp. 333–46.

Olesen, A.B., et al., 2003, Atopic dermatitis is increased following vaccination for measles, mumps and rubella or measles infection, *Acta Dermato-Venereologica*, vol. 83, pp. 445–50.

Onyema, O.O., et al., 2006, Effect of vitamin E on monosodium glutamate induced hepatotoxicity and oxidative stress in rats, *Indian Journal of Biochemistry and Biophysics*, vol. 43, pp. 20–24.

Ordovas, J.M. and Corella, D., 2004, Nutritional genomics, *Annual Reviews of Genomics and Human Genetics*, vol. 5, pp. 71–118.

Palmer, C.N.A., et al., 2006, Common loss-of-function variants of the epidermal barrier protein filaggrin are a major predisposing factor for atopic dermatitis, *Nature Genetics*, vol. 38, no. 4, pp. 441–46.

Penders, J., et al., 2007, Gut microbiota composition and development of atopic manifestations in infancy: the KOALA Birth Cohort Study, *GUT*, vol. 56, no. 5, pp. 661–67.

Pickering L.K. (ed.), 2003, *Red Book: 2003 Report of the Committee on Infectious Diseases*, 26th edition, Elk Grove Village, Ill: American Academy of Pediatrics.

Pike, M.G., et al., 1986, Increased intestinal permeability in atopic eczema, *Journal of Investigative Dermatology*, vol. 86, pp. 101–04.

Popovich, D., et al., 2009, Scurvy forgotten but definitely not gone, *Journal of Pediatric Health Care*, vol. 23, no. 6, pp. 405–15.

Proudfoot, A.T., et al., 2004, Position paper on urine alkalinization, *Clinical Toxicology*, vol. 42, no. 1, pp. 1–26.

Randolf, B.S., et al., 2008, Atopic dermatitis: the role of fungi, *Textbook of Atopic Dermatitis*, Chapter 7, Reitamo, S., Luger, T.A. & Steinhoff, M. (eds), Informa Healthcare, London.

Reitamo, S., et al., 2008, Possible clinical associations of atopic dermatitis with bronchial asthma, *Textbook of Atopic Dermatitis*, Chapter 8, Reitamo, S., Luger, T.A. and Steinhoff, M. (eds), Informa Healthcare, London.

Reitamo, S., Luger, T.A., and Steinhoff, M. (eds), 2008, *Textbook of Atopic Dermatitis*, Informa Healthcare, London.

Rich, A.C., 13 May 1882, On the treatment of eczema by diet, *British Medical Journal*, pp. 695–96.

Richelle, M., et al., 2006, Skin bioavailability of dietary vitamin E, caroteniods, polyphenols, vitamin C, zinc and selenium, *British Journal of Nutrition*, vol. 96, pp. 227–38.

Rosenfeldt V., et al., 2003, Effect of probiotic Lactobacillus strains in children with atopic dermatitis, *Journal of Allergy and Clinical Immunology*, vol. 111, pp. 389–95.

Roth, K.S., 1981, Biotin in clinical medicine — a review, *American Journal of Clinical Nutrition*, vol. 34, pp. 1967–74.

Rudzeviciene, O., et al., 2004, Lactose malabsorption in young Lithuanian children with atopic dermatitis, *Acta Paediatrica*, vol. 93, no. 4, pp. 482–86.

Sampson, H.A. and Jolie, P.L., 1984, Increased plasma histamine concentrations after food challenges in children with atopic dermatitis, *New England Journal of Medicine*, vol. 311, pp. 372–76.

Sariachvili, M., et al., 2010, Early exposure to solid foods and the development of eczema in children up to 4 years of age, *Pediatric Allergy and Immunology*, vol. 21, no. 1 (part 1), pp. 74–81.

Sausenthaler, S., et al., 2006, Margarine and butter consumption, eczema and allergic sensitisation in children, *Pediatric Allergy and Immunology*, vol. 17, no. 2, pp. 85–93.

Sausenthaler, S., et al., 2007, Maternal diet during pregnancy in relation to eczema and allergic sensitisation in the offspring at 2 years of age, *American Journal of Clinical Nutrition*, vol. 85, pp. 530–37.

Savolainen, J., et al., 1993, Candida albicans and atopic dermatitis, *Clinical and Experimental Allergy*, vol. 23, no. 4, pp. 332–39.

Schlueter, A.K. and Johnston, C.S., 2011, Vitamin C: overview and update, *Journal of Evidence-Based Complementary & Alternative Medicine*, vol. 16, no. 49, pp. 49–55.

Schor, J., 2010, Emotions and health: laughter really is good medicine, *Natural Medicine Journal*, vol. 2, no. 1, pp. 1–4.

Sebastian, A., et al., 2002, Estimation of the net acid load of the diet of ancestral preagricultural Homo sapiens and their hominid ancestors, *American Journal of Clinical Nutrition*, vol. 76, pp. 1308–16.

Sicherer, S.H., et al., 1999, Food hyper-sensitivity and atopic dermatitis: pathophysiology, epidemiology, diagnosis and management, *Journal of Allergy & Clinical Immunology*, vol. 104, no. 3, pp. S114–22.

Sidbury, R., et al., 2008, Randomised controlled trial of vitamin D supplementation for winter–related atopic dermatitis in Boston: a pilot study, *British Journal of Dermatology*, vol. 159, pp. 245–46.

Smith, R.L. and Williams, R.T., 1970, History of the discovery of the conjugation mechanisms, pp. 1–19, *Metabolic Conjugation and Metabolic Hydrolysis*, Fishman, W.H. (ed.), Academic Press, New York.

Staberg, B., et al., 1987, Abnormal vitamin D metabolism in patients with psoriasis, *Acta Dermato-Venereologica*, vol. 67, no. 1, abstract, retrieved 22 August 2006: www.ncbi.nlm.nih.gov/sites/entrez

Stanton, R., 2007, *Rosemary Stanton's Complete Book of Food and Nutrition*, Simon & Schuster.

Su, J., 2006, The skin barrier Q&A with dermatologist Dr John Su, Royal Children's Hospital Melbourne, *Eczema Association of Australasia*, retrieved 12 August 2010: www.eczema.org.au/

Sure, B. and Ford, Z.W., 1942, The influence of thiamine, riboflavin, pyridoxine and pantothenic acid deficiencies on nitrogen metabolism, *Journal of Nutrition*, vol. 24, no. 5, pp. 405–26.

Sydenstricker, V.P., et al., 1942, Observations on the egg white injury in man and its cure with a biotin concentrate, *Journal of the American Medical Association*, vol. 118, no. 14, pp. 1199–200.

Thiele, J.J. and Ekanayake-Mudiyanselage, S., 2007, Vitamin E in human skin: organ-specific physiology and considerations for its use in dermatology, *Molecular Aspects of Medicine*, vol. 28, pp. 646–67.

Tsoureli-Nikita, E., Hercogova, J., Lotti, T., and Menchini, G., 2002, Evaluation of dietary intake of vitamin E in the treatment of atopic dermatitis: a study of the clinical course and evaluation of the immunoglobulin E serum levels, *International Journal of Dermatology*, vol. 41, no. 3, pp. 146–50.

Uenishi, T., Sugiura, H., and Uehara, M., 2003, Role of foods in irregular aggravation of atopic dermatitis, *Journal of Dermatology*, vol. 30, pp. 91–97.

Warner J.O., 2001, ETAC Study Group, Early treatment of atopic child. A double-blinded, randomized, placebo-controlled trial of cetirizine in preventing the onset of asthma in children with atopic dermatitis: 18 months' treatment and 18 months' post-treatment follow-up, *Journal of Allergy & Clinical Immunology*, vol. 108, pp. 929–37.

West, C.E., et al., 2009, Probiotics during weaning reduce the incidence of eczema, *Pediatric Allergy and Immunology*, vol. 20, no. 5, pp. 430–37.

Worm, M., et al., 2009, Exogenous histamine aggravates eczema in a subgroup of patients with atopic dermatitis, *Acta Dermato-Venereologica*, vol. 89, pp. 52–6.

Library and Archives Canada Cataloguing in Publication

Fischer, Karen, 1972-, author
      The eczema diet : discover how to stop & prevent the itch of eczema through
      diet & nutrition / Karen Fischer.

Includes index.
ISBN 978-0-7788-0461-1 (pbk.)

      1. Eczema—Diet therapy—Recipes. 2. Eczema—Alternative treatment. I. Title.

RL251.F58 2013   616.5'1   C2013-902504-9

Index

tomato sauce, 168
toners (skin), 132
total daily intake, 98
trans fats, 45
treat days, 155

V

vaccinations, 159
vegans, 14, 156
vegetables, 174–76
  for children, 150, 152
  eczema-safe, 91
  in stage 2, 168–69
vegetables (as ingredient). *See also
    specific vegetables*
  Chickpea Casserole, 224
  Teething Rusks (variation), 204
vegetarians, 14, 156, 169
ventilation, 138
vinegar, apple cider, 172
  Omega Salad Dressing, 220
vinegar, cleaning with, 138
vitamin A, 124
vitamin B_6, 102–3

vitamin C (ascorbic acid), 96–98, 159
  deficiency symptoms, 96
vitamin D, 109–11
vitamin E, 111–13, 130
  for cradle cap, 143

W

washes, 131
water sterilization, 148
wheat, 173
The Wishing Plate, 245
worms, 44

Y

yeasts
  in diet, 41
  as infection cause, 41–43, 45
  on scalp (malassezia), 141
yogurt, 173

Z

zinc, 104–7
  deficiency test, 106

More Great Books
from Robert Rose

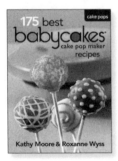

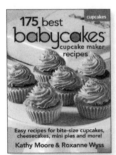

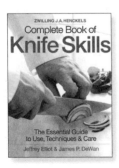

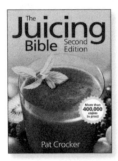

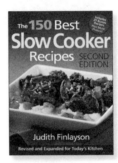

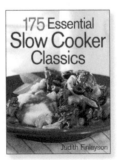

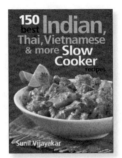

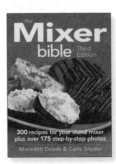

Bestsellers

- The Juicing Bible, Second Edition
  by Pat Crocker
- 175 Best Babycakes™ Cupcake Maker Recipes
  by Kathy Moore and Roxanne Wyss
- 175 Best Babycakes™ Cake Pop Maker Recipes
  by Kathy Moore and Roxanne Wyss
- Eat Raw, Eat Well
  by Douglas McNish
- The Smoothies Bible, Second Edition
  by Pat Crocker
- The Food Substitutions Bible, Second Edition
  by David Joachim
- Zwilling J.A. Henckels Complete Book of Knife Skills
  by Jeffrey Elliot and James P. DeWan

Appliance Bestsellers

- 225 Best Pressure Cooker Recipes
  by Cinda Chavich
- 200 Best Panini Recipes
  by Tiffany Collins
- 125 Best Indoor Grill Recipes
  by Ilana Simon
- The Convection Oven Bible
  by Linda Stephen
- The Fondue Bible
  by Ilana Simon

- 150 Best Indian, Thai, Vietnamese & More Slow Cooker Recipes
  by Sunil Vijayakar
- The 150 Best Slow Cooker Recipes, Second Edition
  by Judith Finlayson
- The Vegetarian Slow Cooker
  by Judith Finlayson
- 175 Essential Slow Cooker Classics
  by Judith Finlayson
- The Healthy Slow Cooker
  by Judith Finlayson
- Slow Cooker Winners
  by Donna-Marie Pye
- Canada's Slow Cooker Winners
  by Donna-Marie Pye
- 300 Best Rice Cooker Recipes
  by Katie Chin
- 650 Best Food Processor Recipes
  by George Geary and Judith Finlayson
- The Mixer Bible, Third Edition
  by Meredith Deeds and Carla Snyder
- 300 Best Bread Machine Recipes
  by Donna Washburn and Heather Butt
- 300 Best Canadian Bread Machine Recipes
  by Donna Washburn and Heather Butt

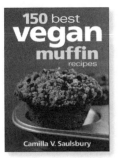

Baking Bestsellers

- 150 Best Gluten-Free Muffin Recipes
  by Camilla V. Saulsbury
- 150 Best Vegan Muffin Recipes
  by Camilla V. Saulsbury
- Piece of Cake!
  by Camilla V. Saulsbury
- 400 Sensational Cookies
  by Linda J. Amendt
- Complete Cake Mix Magic
  by Jill Snider
- 750 Best Muffin Recipes
  by Camilla V. Saulsbury
- 200 Fast & Easy Artisan Breads
  by Judith Fertig

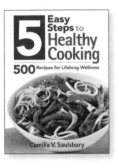

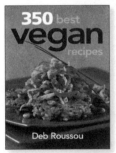
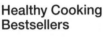

Healthy Cooking Bestsellers

- Canada's Diabetes Meals for Good Health, Second Edition
  by Karen Graham
- Diabetes Meals for Good Health, Second Edition
  by Karen Graham
- 5 Easy Steps to Healthy Cooking
  by Camilla V. Saulsbury
- 350 Best Vegan Recipes
  by Deb Roussou
- The Vegan Cook's Bible
  by Pat Crocker
- The Gluten-Free Baking Book
  by Donna Washburn and Heather Butt

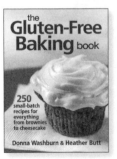

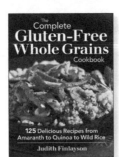

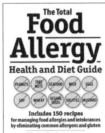
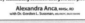

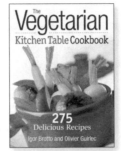

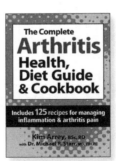

- Complete Gluten-Free Cookbook
  by Donna Washburn and Heather Butt
- 250 Gluten-Free Favorites
  by Donna Washburn and Heather Butt
- Complete Gluten-Free Diet & Nutrition Guide
  by Alexandra Anca and Theresa Santandrea-Cull
- The Complete Gluten-Free Whole Grains Cookbook
  by Judith Finlayson
- The Vegetarian Kitchen Table Cookbook
  by Igor Brotto and Olivier Guiriec

Health Bestsellers

- The Total Food Allergy Health and Diet Guide
  by Alexandra Anca with Dr. Gordon L. Sussman
- The Complete Arthritis Health, Diet Guide & Cookbook
  by Kim Arrey with Dr. Michael R. Starr
- The Essential Cancer Treatment Nutrition Guide & Cookbook
  by Jean LaMantia with Dr. Neil Berinstein
- The Complete Weight-Loss Surgery Guide & Diet Program
  by Sue Ekserci with Dr. Laz Klein
- The PCOS Health & Nutrition Guide
  by Dr. Jillian Stansbury with Dr. Sheila Mitchell

Also Available

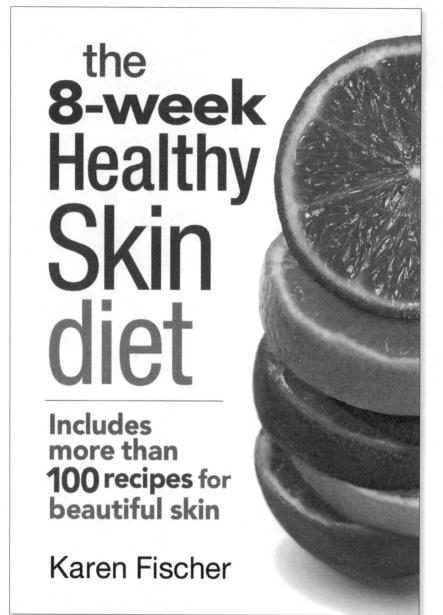

the 8-week Healthy Skin diet

Includes more than **100** recipes for beautiful skin

Karen Fischer

ISBN 978-0-7788-0440-6

Visit us at www.robertrose.ca